Color Atlas of ENT Diagnosis

Tony R. Bull, FRCS
Honorary Consultant Surgeon
Royal National Throat, Nose, and Ear Hospital;
Honorary Senior Lecturer to the Institute of Laryngology and Otology;
Honorary Consultant Surgeon
Charing Cross Hospital;
Consultant Surgeon
King Edward VII Hospital;
London, United Kingdom

John Almeyda, FRCS
Consultant ENT Surgeon
West Middlesex University Hospital
Isleworth, Middlesex
United Kingdom

637 illustrations

5th edition

Thieme
Stuttgart · New York

Library of Congress Cataloging-in-Publication Data is available from the publisher.

Bull, T.R.
   Color atlas of ENT diagnosis / Tony R. Bull, John S. Almeyda. – 5th ed.
   p. ; cm. – (Thieme flexibook)
   Includes index.
   ISBN 978-3-13-129395-4
   1. Otolaryngology–Atlases. 2. Otolaryngology–Diagnosis. I. Almeyda, John S. II. Title. III. Title: ENT diagnosis. IV. Series: Thieme flexibook.
   [DNLM: 1. Otorhinolaryngologic Diseaes–diagnosis–Atlases. WV 17 B935c 2009]
   RF81.B85 2009
   616.2'1075–dc22
                                        2009026131

Illustrations by Roland Geyer, Weilerswist, Germany

© 2010 Georg Thieme Verlag,
Rüdigerstrasse 14, 70469 Stuttgart, Germany
http://www.thieme.de
Thieme New York, 333 Seventh Avenue,
New York, NY 10001, USA
http://www.thieme.com

Cover design: Thieme Publishing Group
Typesetting by Sommer Druck, Feuchtwangen, Germany
Printed in India by Gopsons Paper Limited, New Delhi

ISBN 978-3-13-129395-4

1 2 3 4 5 6

Important note: Medicine is an ever-changing science undergoing continual development. Research and clinical experience are continually expanding our knowledge, in particular our knowledge of proper treatment and drug therapy. Insofar as this book mentions any dosage or application, readers may rest assured that the authors, editors, and publishers have made every effort to ensure that such references are in accordance with **the state of knowledge at the time of production of the book.**

Nevertheless, this does not involve, imply, or express any guarantee or responsibility on the part of the publishers in respect to any dosage instructions and forms of applications stated in the book. **Every user is requested to examine carefully** the manufacturers' leaflets accompanying each drug and to check, if necessary in consultation with a physician or specialist, whether the dosage schedules mentioned therein or the contraindications stated by the manufacturers differ from the statements made in the present book. Such examination is particularly important with drugs that are either rarely used or have been newly released on the market. Every dosage schedule or every form of application used is entirely at the user's own risk and responsibility. The authors and publishers request every user to report to the publishers any discrepancies or inaccuracies noticed. If errors in this work are found after publication, errata will be posted at www.thieme.com on the product description page.

Preface to the 5th edition

Seven years have passed since the previous publication of Color Atlas of ENT Diagnosis and developments in the specialty call for an updated and revised edition. The format of this book remains a pictorial survey of ear, nose, and throat conditions, combined with a succinct text that aims to be of practical help in diagnosis. It is not an illustrated textbook, and further reference is required for more information on the conditions presented. This atlas will, I hope, continue to stimulate the interest of medical students in the specialty and provide useful information to ENT trainees.

In many medical schools ENT undergraduate training is limited. This book will serve as a teaching supplement for medical students, and will also be of practical use to those in general practice and Accident and Emergency departments where ENT conditions are seen so frequently.

T R Bull, FRCS, London
J S Almeyda, FRCS, London

Acknowledgments

Many of the photographs in this book were taken by the authors, but we are grateful for the expertise of the Photographic Departments of the Royal National Throat, Nose and Ear Hospital and the West Middlesex Hospital for many of the better illustrations. Our thanks also go to colleagues who have contributed illustrations to this edition: Professor Lund, Mr Croft, Mr Nasser, Mr Gault, Mr Bailey, Mr Howard, Professor Ramsden, Mr Proops, Professor Weerda, Professor Wright, Dr Glyn Lloyd, Dr AH Davies, Dr Van Hasselt, Dr J Brennand, Dr G Scadding, Professor S. Saieed, Mr Hartley, and Mr Peter Bull.

Figure 4.**64** has been reprinted with permission from: Farthing CF, Brown SE, Color Atlas of Aids and HIV Disease, 2nd edition, 1998, Mosby Wolfe, London.

We also thank the audiologist, Mr Ganguly, for his advice on the audiometry section.

Contents

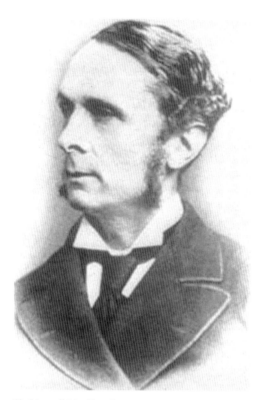

Sir Morrell MacKenzie

The Scottish physician and surgeon who founded Ear, Nose, and Throat as a specialty and wrote the first standard textbook on Rhinology and Laryngology. Sir Morrell MacKenzie also founded one of the first hospitals for nose and throat diseases in London in 1863 (today the Royal National Throat, Nose and Ear Hospital). The most common condition he treated in this hospital was laryngeal tuberculosis, at that time invariably fatal, but today uncommon and curable.

1 ENT Examination

Instruments

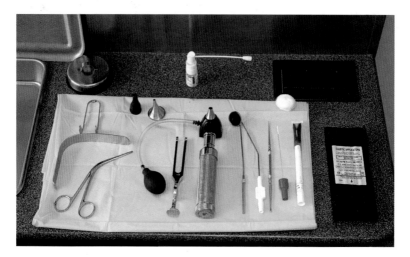

Fig. 1.1 **The instruments needed for an ENT examination:** The *laryngeal and postnasal mirrors* require warming to avoid misting, and hot water or a spirit lamp is necessary. An angled *tongue depressor* or wooden spatula is needed for examining the oropharynx and postnasal space. *Angled forceps* are used for dressing the nose or ear. A *tuning fork* is essential for the diagnosis of conductive or sensorineural (perceptive) hearing loss. A C1 or C2 (256 or 512 cps) is needed. The very large tuning forks used to test vibration sense are unsatisfactory, and may give a false Rinne test. A *Jobson-Horne probe* is widely used in ENT departments. A loop on one end is for removing wax (and foreign bodies) from the ear or nose. Cotton wool attached to the other end is used for cleaning the ear.

An *auriscope, nasal* and *aural specula* complete the basic instruments. A *sterile swab* and *media* are necessary for throat, nasal, or ear specimens to be taken for culture and sensitivity. A "narrow" swab holder as shown here is extremely useful for aural specimens, as the more common swab is too wide and can be traumatic for the deep meatus and middle ear.

The doctor's clean white coat remains appropriate dress for noninterventional examination when using these instruments. Surveys have shown that patients prefer their doctor not to wear casual dress. "Scrubs" are frequently used now for patient examination and are necessary for interventional procedures. The concern of cross infection has led to the use of disposable instruments, but this is not at present established practice.

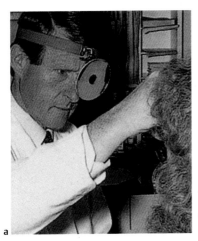
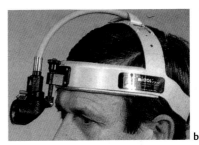

a
b

Fig. 1.**2a, b Lighting.** The *head mirror* (**a**) gives effective lighting for examining the upper respiratory tract and ear, and leaves both hands free for using the instruments. Initially, the technique of using a head mirror is not easy, and some may prefer a *fiberoptic* or *electric headlight* (**b**).

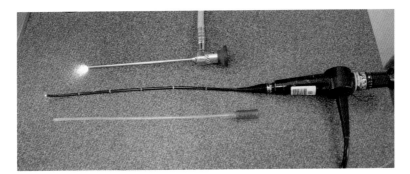

Fig. 1.**3 Rigid and flexible fiberoptic endoscopes.** These are important additional examination instruments. The flexible endoscope is of value to see the laryngeal region (see Fig. 1.**61**) in those with a marked gag reflex in whom indirect laryngoscopy (see Fig. 1.**60**) with a mirror is difficult. The rigid endoscope is important in examination of the nasal cavities.

A sterile plastic sheath to use over the endoscope is also shown.

Examination of the Ear

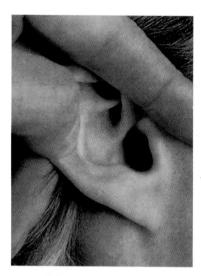

Fig. 1.**4 Retracting the pinna.** The meatus is S-shaped. To see the drum more clearly, therefore, the pinna is retracted backwards and outwards. The index finger may be used to hold the tragus forward. If this step of straightening the meatus accentuates the pain in someone presenting with an earache, one can be virtually certain that the diagnosis is either a furuncle or furunculosis (see Fig. 2.**47**).

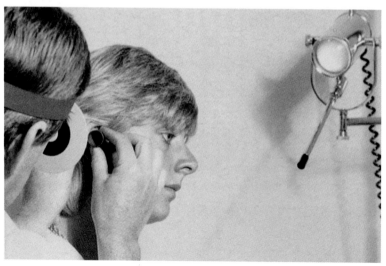

Fig. 1.**5 Head mirror and speculum.** These are used for the initial examination of the meatus and drum.

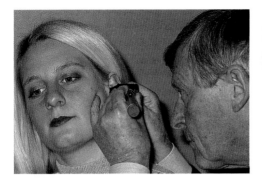

Fig. 1.**6 The auriscope.** This is ***best held like a pen.*** In this way, the examiner's little finger can rest on the patient's cheek; if the patient's head moves, the position of the ear speculum is maintained in the meatus.

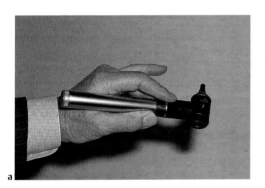

Fig. 1.**7a Preferred way to hold the auriscope.** When the left ear is examined, the auriscope is held in the left hand and vice versa.

a

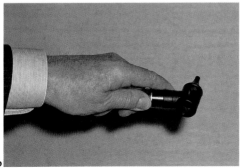

b Incorrect way to hold the auriscope.

b

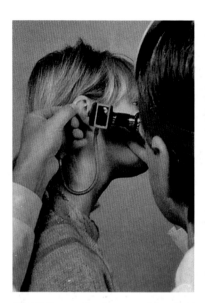

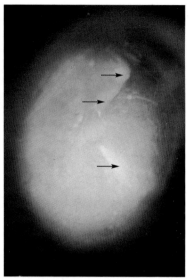

Fig. 1.8 Pneumatic otoscope. A handheld air-filled bulb attached to the auriscope enables air to be gently inflated against the drum to demonstrate drum mobility.

Reduced mobility is conspicuous and is *evidence of middle ear fluid*. Reduced mobility is also seen, however, with tympanosclerosis, which increases the rigidity of the drum. Malleus fixation is a rare cause of reduced mobility of a drum of normal appearance.

The *fistula test* may be done with the pneumatic otoscope. Pressure change by pressing on the bulb will cause dizziness in those with erosion of the labyrinth by *cholesteatoma* (see Fig. 2.**68**) or with a *perilymph fistula*.

Fig. 1.9 A normal drum. The *main landmarks* seen on the pars tensa of a normal drum are the *lateral process* (top arrow) and *handle* (middle arrow) of the *malleus*, and the *light reflex* (lower arrow). The drum superior to the short process is the pars flaccida or attic part of the drum. A normal drum is grey and varies in vascularity and translucency.

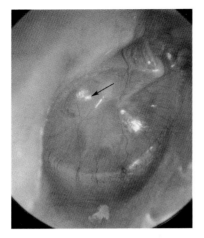

Fig. 1.**10 A tympanic membrane showing the panoramic view obtained with a fiberoptic endoscope.** Fiberoptic auriscopes are not in common use and the conventional auriscope is widely used. For this reason most drums are shown as they are seen with an auriscope. It is interesting to compare the appearance of a normal drum with the auriscope and the appearance with a fiberoptic. A thin posterior scar indrawn onto the stapes is clearly seen (arrow) and would not be so apparent with most conventional auriscopes.

For the most clear view of the eardrum, and for fine use of instruments, the microscope (Fig. 1.**15**) is used.

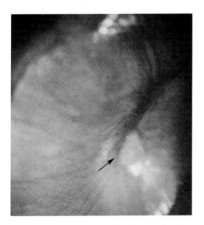

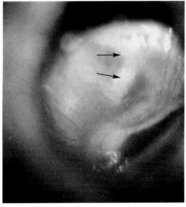

Fig. 1.**11 A more vascular drum.** This has vessels extending down the handle of the malleus to the umbo (arrow).

These vessels may also be more conspicuous following mild barotrauma to the ear, e.g., rapid descent in an airplane in which delayed eustachian tube opening causes pain. More severe trauma leads to hemorrhage into the drum or perforation.

Fig. 1.**12 The incus** (lower arrow) **may show as a shadow through a thin drum,** as may the round window and opening of the eustachian tube, although this is less common. The chorda tympani nerve may also be seen through the drum (top arrow).

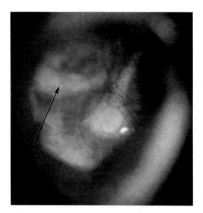

Fig. 1.**13 The chorda tympani nerve** is the nerve of taste to the anterior two thirds of the tongue (excluding the circumvallate papillae), and is also the secretomotor nerve to the submandibular and sublingual salivary glands. The chorda tympani nerve usually lies behind the pars flaccida. It is not normally visible, but if the nerve is more inferior, it shows through the drum (arrow).

Referred Ear Pain

If examination of the drum and meatus is normal in a patient complaining of earache, the pain is referred. **_Referred ear pain_** may be from nearby structures such as the temporo-mandibular joint, neck muscles, or cervical spine. It may also be from the teeth, tongue, tonsils, or larynx. Cranial nerves V, IX, and X which supply these sites have their respective tympanic and auricular branches supplying the ear. Earache also frequently precedes a Bell's palsy.

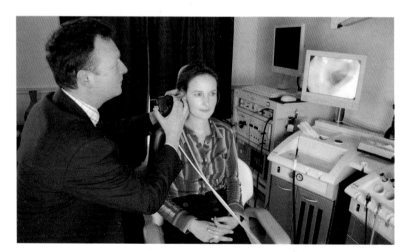

Fig. 1.**14 Examination of the ear with an otoendoscope or microscope** when projected to a TV monitor is a useful teaching aid and a reassurance to some patients.

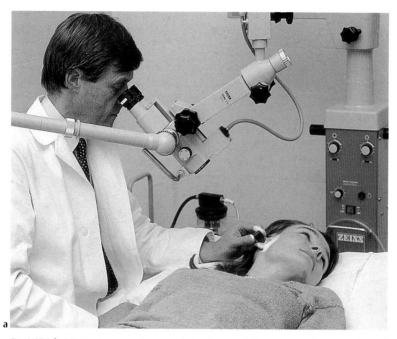

Fig. 1.15a, b Microscope examination of the drum. a Although most drums can be well seen and conditions diagnosed with the auriscope, the increased magnification that is obtainable with the operating microscope and easier instrumentation, make this apparatus standard in any well-equipped outpatient department. A video camera or tutor arm may be attached to the microscope for demonstration. The auricular branch of the vagus nerve sup-

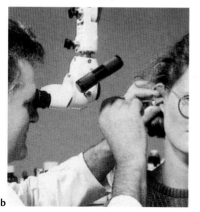

plies part of the deep meatus and eardrum, as well as some skin in the post auricular fold. Therefore, instrumentation of the ear may produce a sensation of faintness from a vasovagal episode; also a cough may be triggered. Many therefore prefer to have the ear examination with the patient lying down, particularly for procedures such as difficult suction clearance of wax and debris from the deep meatus. Routine examination of the drum with the microscope may be carried out with the patient sitting up (**b**).

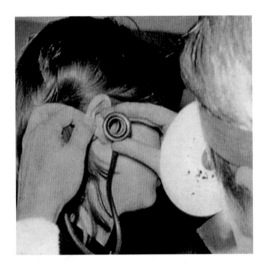

Fig. 1.**16**   **Siegle's speculum.** The pneumatic otoscope has replaced the use of Siegle's speculum (see Fig. 1.**8**). With plain (not magnifying) glass it is useful to test drum mobility with the microscope.

Hearing Loss

Most hearing loss is easy to diagnose as either a well-defined **conductive or sensorineural type**. ("Mixed" hearing loss may occur, but this diagnosis is usually non-contributory, and the term is better avoided.)

Lesions to the left of the red line (Fig. 1.**17**) cause **conductive** hearing loss, and are frequently curable. Hearing loss to the right of the red line is due to a **sensorineural** lesion, and is usually not so amenable to treatment. The black line separates the cochlear from the retrocochlear hearing losses.

The etiology and management of "sudden" sensorineural hearing loss remains controversial. Etiological factors include viral infections, vascular occlusion, an autoimmune process or membrane breaks. Discussion of the treatment, both conservative and interventional (steroids orally or intratympanically) is of importance as spontaneous hearing improvement is common.

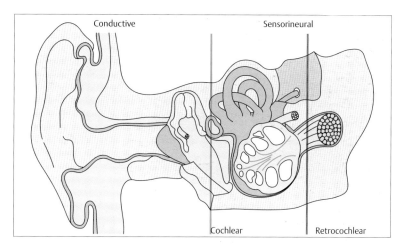

Fig. 1.**17 Conductive and sensorineural hearing loss.** *Hearing loss is either conductive or sensorineural in type. It is an essential basic step in diagnosis of hearing loss to distinguish between these two.* Sensorineural hearing loss is either due to a cochlear or retrocochlear lesion.

Tests for Conductive and Sensorineural Hearing Loss

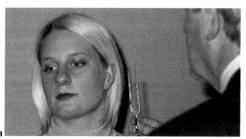

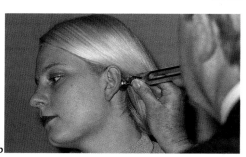

Fig. 1.**18a, b The Rinne test.** *Tuning fork tests are essential preliminary tests for the diagnosis of hearing loss.*

The Rinne and Weber tests enable the diagnosis of a conductive or sensorineural hearing loss to be made. If the tuning fork is heard louder on the mastoid process than in front of the ear, the Rinne test is negative, and the hearing loss conductive. If the tuning fork is heard better in front of the ear, the Rinne test is positive, and the hearing is either normal or there is sensorineural hearing loss.

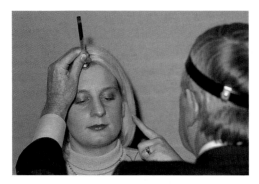

Fig. 1.**19 The Weber test.** The tuning fork, when held in the mid-line on the forehead, is heard in the ear with the conductive hearing loss. This test is very sensitive, and if the meatus is occluded with the finger, the tuning fork will be heard in that ear. A conductive loss of as little as 5 dB will result in the Weber test being referred to that ear.

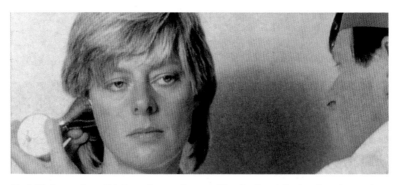

Fig. 1.**20 Barany box.** This is used to *confirm total hearing loss.* It is placed on the good ear and produces a noise totally masking this ear. The patient will be unable to repeat words clearly spoken into the deaf ear.

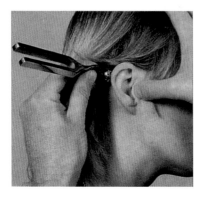

Fig. 1.**21 The occlusion (Bing).** This is also helpful. The tuning fork is held on the mastoid process and the tragus lightly pushed to occlude the meatus. The tuning fork is heard louder, in conductive hearing loss, even of a slight degree, there is no change when the meatus is occluded. The Rinne test does not become negative until there is a marked degree of conductive loss (about a 20-dB air–bone gap). It is therefore possible to have a slight conductive hearing loss with a positive Rinne test. The more sensitive occlusion test will help in the diagnosis.

Total Hearing Loss in One Ear

Total hearing loss in one ear is frequently wrongly diagnosed as a conductive hearing loss. The Rinne is negative because the tuning fork, although not heard in front of the ear, is heard by the better ear when placed on the mastoid process of the deaf ear, with the sound being transmitted by the bone (false-negative Rinne). The Weber test gives the clue that the Rinne is false, as the sound will not lateralize to the deaf ear.

Total hearing loss in one ear may be congenital or the result of a skull fracture. Meningitis is also a cause, but ***mumps*** is probably the commonest cause, and an ***acoustic neuroma*** must be excluded.

Hearing Aids

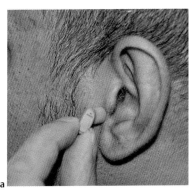

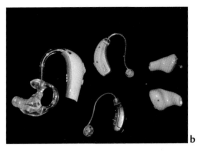

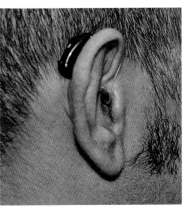

Fig. 1.**22a–c Digital hearing aids. a** *In the ear* (ITE) digital hearing aids fit neatly into the ear canal and are suitable for mild to moderately severe hearing loss.

b Examples of modern hearing aids. Modern digital hearing aids are fully automatic and improve speech intelligibility in background noise by using directional microphones and compression technology.

c *Receiver in the ear canal* (RIC) digital hearing aids. These are for mild to moderate sensorineural hearing loss. A receiver placed in the ear canal is attached by a thin wire to the postaural hearing aid, so keeping the ear canal "open." This prevents the "occlusion effect" and preserves natural low frequency hearing.

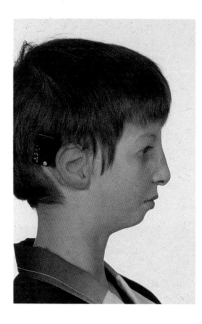

Fig. 1.**23 Bone-anchored hearing aid.** The aid clips onto osseo-integrated titanium screws fixed to the mastoid bone. It is an efficient sound conductor for those with congenital absence or deformity of the ear canal and pinna, in whom a conventional hearing aid cannot be fitted.

With ear discharge not controlled medically or surgically, the fitting of a conventional aid for conductive hearing loss is also not practical, and bone-anchored aids may be used.

Fig. 1.**24a–f The cochlear implant** has proved a great advance in the management of profound hearing loss in children and adults, where conventional aids are ineffective for hearing restoration.

a, b Cochlear implant incision: The incision takes into account the proposed position of the implanted receiver–stimulator package and the external ear-level processor.

c An ear-level microphone is fitted like a hearing aid. Sound is converted to electric signals that are sent to a processor and transmitted to electrodes inserted into the cochlear. External components: microphone, speech processor, and induction coil.

d The nuclear contour electrode contains a stylette. When the stylette is removed, the coil forms a curl that conforms to the cochlear.

e The nuclear contour device contains 22 electro-terminals, which can be seen on the radiograph showing the implant in place in the inner ear.

f This image shows the implanted hardware: receiver–stimulator package, active and reference electrodes.

(Images **c**, **d**, **f** courtesy of Cochlear UK, Addlestone, Surrey, UK.)

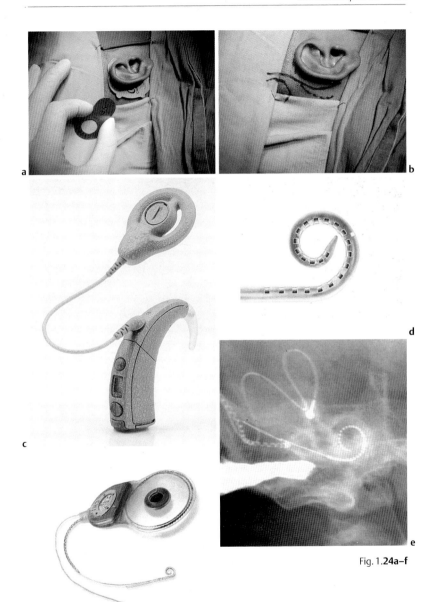

Fig. 1.**24a–f**

Investigation of Hearing Loss: Radiology

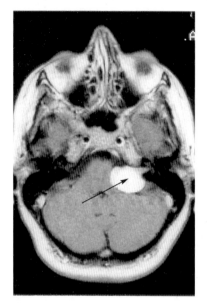

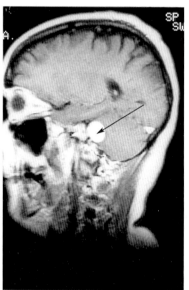

Fig. 1.25 **Acoustic neuroma.** *The most common early presentation of an acoustic neuroma is a unilateral sensorineural hearing loss.* An MRI scan is an essential investigation to exclude this tumor in all cases of unilateral sensorineural hearing loss unless there is a certain other cause, e.g., trauma, mumps, meningitis. There is now a marked awareness that sensorineural loss, particularly if unilateral and even if minimal, requires investigation to exclude an acoustic neuroma.

Fig. 1.26 **The MRI and CT scan** are two important radiograph innovations developed in Great Britain. The MRI scan gives the diagnosis of acoustic neuroma (arrows).

Magnetic resonance imaging is the single most important investigation for acoustic neuroma. Early diagnosis is important for a small neuroma (less than 1 cm in diameter). This can be removed with preservation of the facial nerve to which it is adjacent in the internal auditory meatus, and the hearing too may be preserved.

Neuromas arise from the nerve sheath of the vestibular nerve (strictly termed "schwannomas"), and may be dissected from the auditory nerve. The prognosis for larger neuromas is less good, with risk of permanent damage to the facial nerve and increased morbidity from intracranial surgery.

Surgery remains the mainstay of treatment for vestibular schwannoma. The increased investigation of asymmetric hearing loss by MRI scanning has led to many small tumors being discovered. A "wait and re-scan" approach is appropriate for small intracanalicular tumors as many grow slowly or remain static. Gamma knife stereotactic radio surgery is an alternative treatment modality with high-dose radiation directed precisely to the tumor using a frame fixed to the patient.

Investigation of Hearing Loss: Audiometry

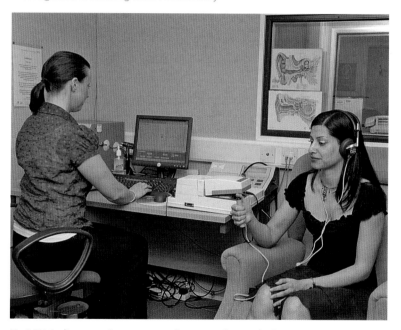

Fig. 1.**27 Audiometry.** A ***pure-tone audiogram*** is the standard test of hearing level. The readings are recorded on a chart with intensity (0–120 dB) and frequency (usually 250–8000 cps). A normal tracing is between –0 dB and +10 dB at all frequencies. This test is accurate to about 10 dB only, as there are variables due to the patient's responses and the accuracy of both the audiometrician and the machine. Hearing is tested in front of the ear (air conduction—recorded in black) and over the mastoid process (bone conduction—recorded in red). A silent or soundproof room is necessary for accurate pure-tone audiometry.

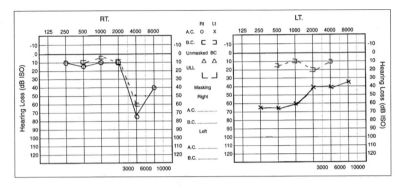

Fig. 1.**28 Audiogram**. The audiogram on the left shows a typical sensorineural hearing loss; a sharp dip at 4000 cps, as on this chart, is typical of inner ear damage due to **noise trauma**. A loss of high frequencies is commonly seen in hearing loss of old age (**presbycusis**). The audiogram on the right shows a conductive hearing loss with the sound heard better on the bone, typical of **otosclerosis** or **otitis media**.

Audiometry requires skill and training, particularly to test children. An audiogram is obtainable from most children by age three to four. With unilateral hearing loss, noise is used to mask the better ear, so that this ear does not hear the sound transmission from the deaf ear and give a false reading. Hearing assessment under the age of three years, or in children who are unable to cooperate with audiometry, requires special skills and techniques.

The response of a baby or toddler to meaningful sounds, such as a spoon "chinked" against a cup, gives an indication of hearing. **Electrocochleography** (ECoG) involves placing fine electrodes through the drum to pick up auditory nerve reaction potential in response to sound. This refined test gives a good hearing assessment for infants in whom a hearing loss is suspected. Anesthesia is required for ECoG. This objective test of hearing acuity is also of help in the diagnosis of psychosomatic hearing loss or malingering. The **auditory brain stem response** (ABR), in which electroencephalogram recordings are made following auditory stimulus, is another useful audiometric test.

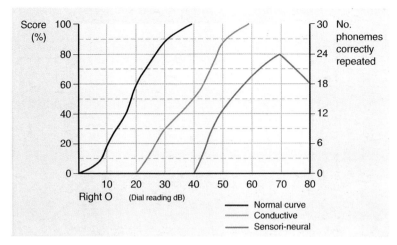

Fig. 1.**29 Speech discrimination audiometry**. A criticism of puretone audiometry is that an assessment of the ability to hear puretone sounds may not reflect the ability to hear speech. A phonetically balanced list of words is used. The percentage of those correctly detected is used as the index to plot a speech discrimination chart. The ability to understand speech is obviously reduced with all hearing loss but particularly with sensorineural loss in which the high tones are involved. An additional help in the diagnosis of acoustic neuromas may be poor speech discrimination, in excess of that expected from the level of the pure-tone audiogram.

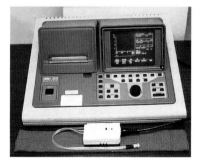

Fig. 1.**30 Impedance audiometry** involves performing several measurements to obtain a wide range of information about the middle and inner ear. A probe with a rubber tip and containing three small patent tubes is fitted into the meatus to make an airtight seal. One tube delivers the tone to the ear, a second tube is attached to a microphone to monitor the sound pressure level within the ear canal, and a third tube is attached to a manometer to vary the air pressure in the ear.

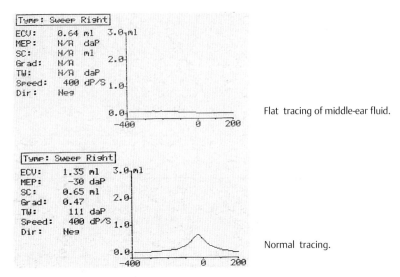

Flat tracing of middle-ear fluid.

Normal tracing.

Fig. 1.**31 Impedance measurements** are particularly helpful in the differential diagnosis of conductive and sensorineural hearing losses, as they give information about middle-ear pressure, eustachian tube function, middle-ear reflexes, and the level of a lower motor neuron facial nerve palsy. *Impedance testing is widely used to confirm the presence of middle-ear fluid, and the "flat" tracing is characteristic.* A "glue ear" may be diagnosed in babies and younger children using impedance measurements when the cooperation required for a pure-tone audiogram is not possible.

Otoacoustic Emissions

In children or babies who are suspected of having a hearing loss who are too young for audiometry, *otoacoustic emissions* (OAEs) give a valuable objective *assessment of hearing.* OAEs are a test of outer hair cell function. Introducing a broad band "click" to the ear causes the cochlear to emit a sound, which can then be amplified and analyzed. Where marked sensorineural loss exists OAEs cannot be detected. This test may also be helpful in the diagnosis of non-organic hearing loss.

Tests of Balance

Vertigo is most commonly due to a disorder of the labyrinth. A sensation of unsteadiness may occur, however, with hypoglycemia, orthostatic hypotension, hyperventilation, and cerebral ischemia. Tumors or multiple sclerosis involving the vestibular system also cause imbalance.

Abnormalities in these preliminary clinical tests of balance will indicate the need for further investigation.

Vertigo due to a labyrinth disorder may occur with or without hearing loss.

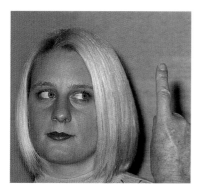

Fig. 1.**32 Observation for nystagmus** is one of the clinical tests for abnormalities of balance. Nystagmus due to a labyrinth disorder is characterized by a slow and quick phase of eye movement in which the eye moves slowly away from the side of the involved labyrinth, then flicks rapidly back to that side; the nystagmus is said to be in the direction of the quick phase. The eye movement in nystagmus is fine.

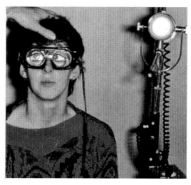

Fig. 1.**33 Frenzel glasses**. Observation of nystagmus is facilitated by fitting the patient with glasses with magnifying lenses, such as Frenzel glasses.

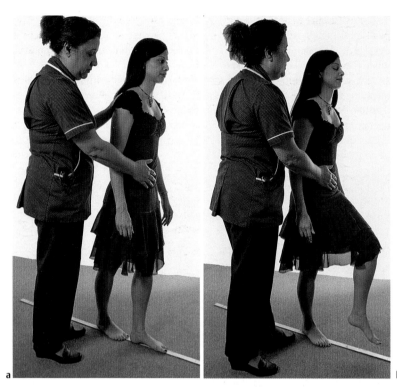

Fig. 1.**34a, b Tests to demonstrate abnormalities of gait. a** One of these is heel-toe walk-ing along a straight line. A person with normal balance is stable without looking down at the feet. **b The Romberg test** is another basic test of balance. This test, in which the patient is asked to stand still with feet together and eyes closed, is made more sensitive by asking the patient to mark time, when instability is obvious, indicating a significant balance dis-order.

Positional Vertigo

Benign paroxysmal positional vertigo is a sudden and severe rotary vertigo occurring when lying down in bed or upon looking upwards, when the head is placed backwards and to one side. There is no hearing loss, and it may follow a head injury. Although common, it is frequently not recognized, and unneces-sary neurological investigation may be carried out.

The positional history is typical, and diagnosis is confirmed by a **positive positional test.** When the head is placed backwards and to one side there is nystagmus which fatigues within several seconds, but recurs temporarily when the patient sits up.

This is a self-limiting condition, and advising the patient simply to avoid the position that triggers off the attack may suffice as treatment. With benign paroxysmal positional vertigo the episodes may vary in severity, duration, and frequency, and also tend to recur. The **Epley maneuver** (Fig. **1.36a–d**) is effective in curtailing benign paroxysmal positional vertigo. The condition is believed to be caused by displaced calcium particles from the utricle forming debris in the semicircular canals of the labyrinth. Head positions of the Epley maneuver aim to reposition these particles in the labyrinth so they do not affect the canal dynamics. Positional vertigo may also occur with space-occupying lesions involving the cerebellum and cerebello-pontine angle. Nystagmus may be induced with the positional test, but there is no latent period and the nystagmus does not fatigue.

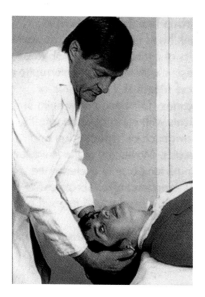

Fig. 1.**35 Positional test for benign paroxysmal positional vertigo.**

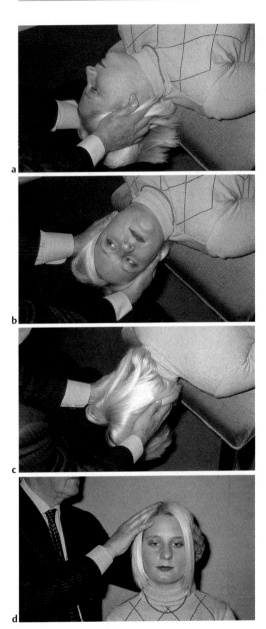

Fig. 1.36a–d The Epley maneuver. The patient lies down with the head in the position to trigger positional vertigo (**a**). After 30–60 seconds, when the nystagmus has settled, the head is turned through 90° to the opposite side (**b**), and remains there for a further minute. The patient is then rolled on to that side with the head maintained in this position, and the head is then rotated so that the patient is facing obliquely downwards for a further minute (**c**). The sitting position is then resumed while maintaining head rotation, and the head is finally rotated to the central position (**d**) and moved 40° downwards to complete the Epley maneuver.

Advice to keep the head erect and avoid the trigger position is given. Three or more pillows are advised when sleeping. The Epley maneuver may be repeated if ineffective in the first instance.

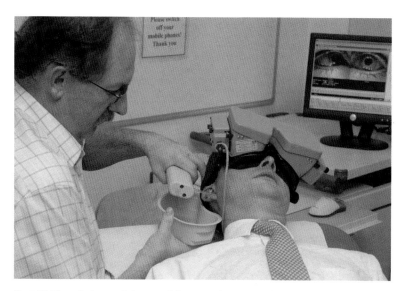

Fig. 1.**37 The caloric test.** Irrigation of the external meatus with water 7° above and later 7° below body temperature sets up convection currents of the endolymph in the semicircular canals. This causes nystagmus, and the duration of the nystagmus gives an index of the activity of the labyrinth. The nystagmus can be directly observed or recorded electrically (***electronystagmography***) or by video nystagmography where small goggle-mounted video cameras obtain images of eye movement. This test is particularly valuable in the diagnosis of Ménière's disease and acoustic neuroma. A reduced or absent nystagmus is found (canal paresis).

Ménière's Disease

Sudden severe rotary vertigo often with nausea and vomiting, a tinnitus increasing prior to the vertigo, and a sensorineural hearing loss (cochlear type), which may fluctuate, form the triad of symptoms characteristic of Ménière's disease.

Distorted hearing (diplacusis) and a sensation of "pressure" in the ear are often further symptoms.

In this curious condition, there is an increase in the endolymph volume, but the cause is unknown. The disease has a reputation for being serious, which is not justified. Although the vertigo may occasionally be severe and incapacitating, the symptoms are frequently mild, usually self-limiting, and not progressive. It is never fatal, and medical treatment with labyrinthine sedatives, for example, prochlorperazine, commonly controls the vertigo. Oral

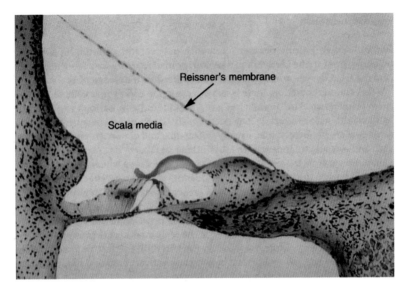

Fig. 1.**38** **Normal ear.**

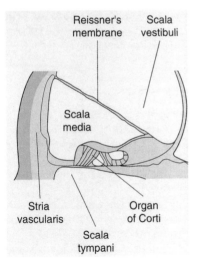

Fig. 1.**39** **Illustration of normal ear.**

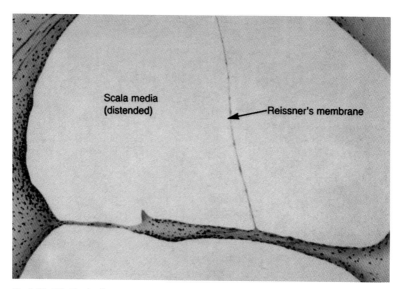

Fig. 1.40 Ménière's disease.

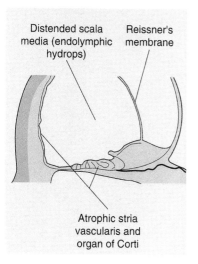

Fig. 1.**41 Illustration of ear with Ménière's disease**, showing atrophic stria vascularis and organ of Corti.

histamine-like drugs which aim to increase the blood flow to the inner ear (e.g., betahistine) may also be effective, as may a low salt diet and diuretics. There is, however, no proven specific medical therapy at present available for Ménière's disease.

In one more recent treatment of Ménière's disease, Gentamycin instilled into the middle ear either directly through the drum or via a catheter, is absorbed through the round window membrane into the inner ear. Gentamycin is more toxic to the vestibular apparatus than the cochlear and the dose can be titrated to destroy vestibular function with minimal effect on the hearing. All patients are, however, warned that there is a risk to hearing with this treatment. Good control rates for vertigo have been reported with the treatment.

Many innovative surgical procedures have been tried for Ménière's disease; none of them has proved to be totally successful, although decompression of the endolymphatic sac in an attempt to reduce the pressure in the scala media may prove effective conservative surgery. Surgery to destroy the labyrinth is effective in controlling the vertigo, but an irreversible total hearing loss with accentuated tinnitus is one of the factors that make this treatment a last resort.

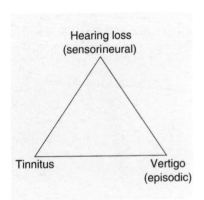

Fig. 1.42 **The triad of Ménière's disease.**

Tinnitus

Tinnitus is commonly associated with hearing loss, although it may rarely be troublesome with normal hearing. Tinnitus with conductive hearing loss is usually less distressing than tinnitus with sensorineural hearing loss, as in the latter the tinnitus may cause serious psychiatric disturbance. The full physiology and pathology of tinnitus remains unknown, and there is no entirely effective treatment. Explanation and reassurance are helpful in the patient's acceptance of tinnitus (patients frequently associate it with serious intracranial disease), and the use of a tranquilizer may be necessary. A tinnitus associated with sensorineural hearing loss is usually a continuous tone (frequently described as "like listening to a sea shell"). Tinnitus may, however, be pulsatile and needs investigation (e.g., computed tomography [CT] or magnetic resonance imaging [MRI] scan), to exclude a vascular lesion, for example, glomus jugulare (Fig. 2.**92**). No cause may be found for pulsatile tinnitus synchronous with the pulse.

In *sound therapy* a hearing aid-like device which generates a noise matched to the patient's tinnitus is fitted to the ear. This noise input acts as a tinnitus masker and is one of the treatments for tinnitus.

On the basis of a neurophysiological model of tinnitus involving abnormal sound processing, *tinnitus retraining therapy* combines sound therapy with cognitive behavioral techniques. Surgical treatment of tinnitus with section of the acoustic nerve or destruction of the inner ear has been tried and is unsatisfactory.

Examination of the Nose

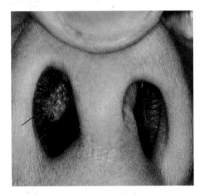

Fig. 1.**43   Examining a child.** Instruments are best avoided in children. A good anterior view of the nose can be obtained simply by pressing on the tip of the nose. In this case, a clear view is obtained of a pedunculated papilloma of the nasal vestibule (arrow).

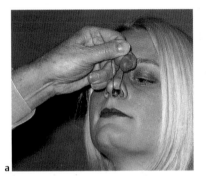

a

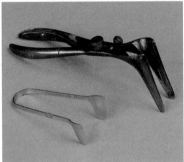

b

Fig. 1.**44a   Speculum examination shows** the nasal vestibule, the septum anteriorly (particularly Little's area—see Fig. 3.**98**), and the inferior and middle turbinates anteriorly. **b** There are several different types of nasal speculum used throughout the world. The ones demonstrated here are Thudicum (left) and the Killian (right) speculums.

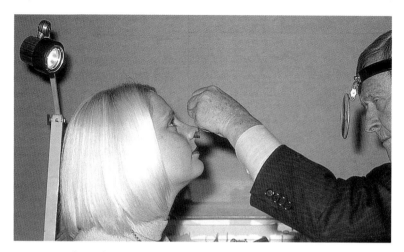

Fig. 1.**45 Nasal speculum examination.**

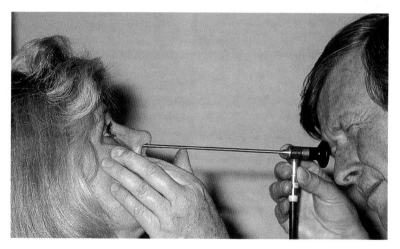

Fig. 1.**46 A nasal endoscope** is necessary for a thorough examination of the nasal cavities, the mucosa having been sprayed with surface anesthetic.

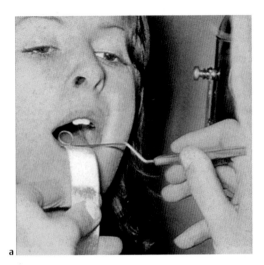

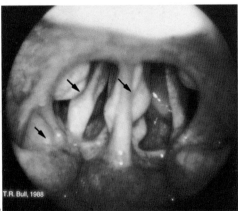

Fig. 1.**47a   Mirror examination of the postnasal space.** This is not easy, particularly in children. With a patient who gags easily, or whose soft palate is close to the posterior wall of the oropharynx, a view may be impossible.

b With a fiberoptic endoscope (see Fig. 1.**46**), however, a clear view of the postnasal space is obtained, and instrumentation for biopsies of the postnasal space via the fiberoptic endoscope are available. The panoramic endoscopic view of the postnasal space obtained per orally demonstrates all anatomical features, but is not often achieved in the outpatient setting.

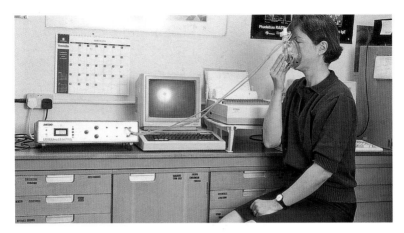

Fig. 1.**48 Rhinomanometry** techniques give a quantitative measurement of nasal airways. Many methods have been employed, but the anterior active method has gained most acceptance. The pressure is measured through one nostril, while the flow is measured through the opposite side using a face mask and pneumotach. Rhinometry has yet to become of sufficient clinical value to be of routine use in the assessment of nasal obstruction, as the threshold of nasal obstruction or "congestion" of which the patient complains correlates poorly with air pressure measurements.

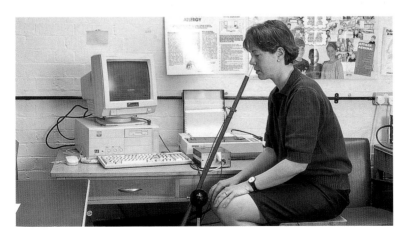

Fig. 1.**49 Acoustic rhinomanometry.** A series of clicks are introduced into the nasal vestibule and reflected from the interior of the nose by the structures within, in a similar fashion to tympanometry. The reflected sounds are captured by a microphone and transformed into a graph of nasal cross-sectional area against distance into the nose.

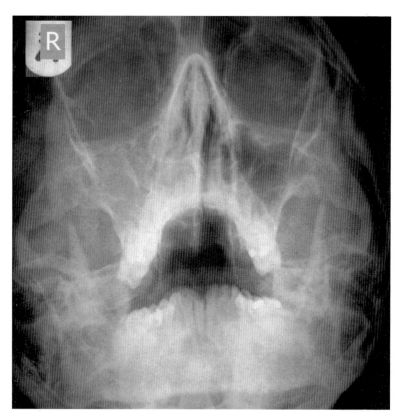

Fig. 1.**50 Sinus radiographs have largely been displaced by CT scans for the investigation of sinus disease.** Plain radiographs are, however, helpful in diagnosis, showing opacity, indicating infection or polyposis and bone expansion or erosion, suggestive of neoplasm. Plain radiographs are also inexpensive and involve minimal radiation compared to CT scans. This X-ray shows opacity of the right maxillary sinus.

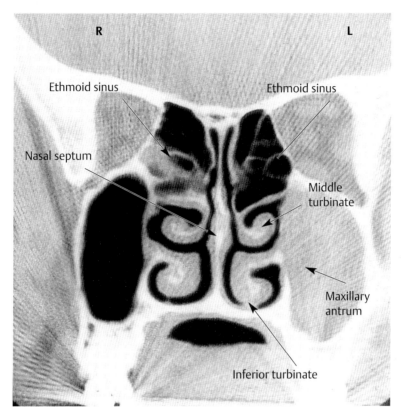

R   **L**

Ethmoid sinus   Ethmoid sinus

Nasal septum

Middle
turbinate

Maxillary
antrum

Inferior turbinate

Fig. 1.**51** **A CT scan of the sinuses** gives precise detail, particularly of the ethmoids, which are not well seen on the plain radiograph. The CT scan is important prior to sinus surgery. The left maxillary antrum is seen to be opaque on this radiograph from infection, but the left ethmoids are clear. Some minimal mucosal thickening (which would not be detected on plain radiographs) is seen in the right ethmoid sinus.

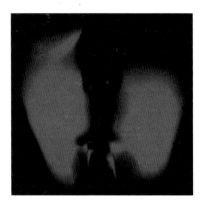

Fig. 1.**52 Transillumination**. A bright light held inside the mouth in a dark room is an investigation very rarely used. A dull antrum is, however, an additional sign in the diagnosis of maxillary sinus disease. Transillumination is useful to assess whether a sinusitis is settling. Dental cysts involving the antrum transilluminate brightly.

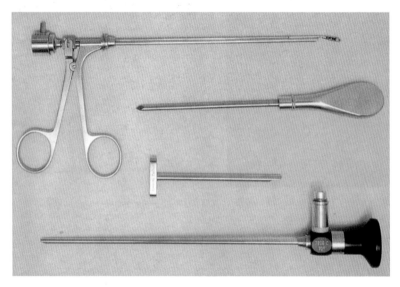

Fig. 1.**53 Sinus endoscopy (antroscopy).** A narrow endoscope inserted into the maxillary antrum, either through the thin bony wall of the canine fossa intraorally or via the inferior meatus of the nasal fossa under the inferior turbinate, gives a good view of the interior of the maxillary sinus, and is helpful in diagnosis.

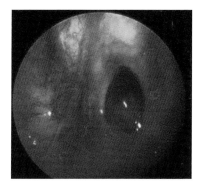

Fig. 1.**54 The ostium of the maxillary sinus** seen through the endoscope.

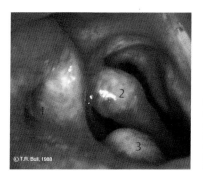

Fig. 1.**55 The postnasal space.** Enlarged view of Fig. 1.**47b** to show the eustachian orifice (1) and posterior ends of the middle (2) and inferior (3) turbinate.

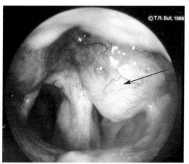

Fig. 1.**56 A postnasal cyst (Thornvaldts, arrow)** demonstrated with a fiberoptic photograph of the postnasal space.

Skin Prick Tests

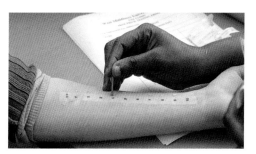

Fig. 1.**57 Skin prick tests.** A series of standardized allergens with positive and negative controls are pricked into the skin using a lancet. The responses are checked at 15 minutes. The tests are immediate and inexpensive, but there is a small risk of anaphylaxis.

Examination of the Pharynx and Larynx

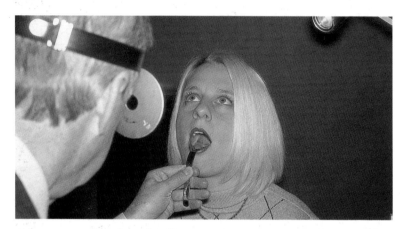

Fig. 1.**58 Examination of the pharynx.** A tongue depressor is necessary to obtain a clear view of the tonsil region in most cases. Patients vary however in how easily the fauces and posterior aspects of the tongue can be seen. On occasion a very clear view is obtained (Fig. 1.**59**).

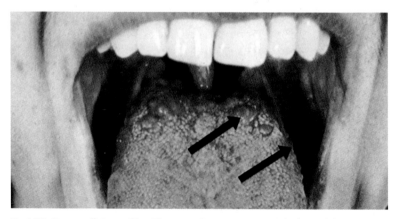

Fig. 1.**59 Circumvallate papillae.** These are often prominent on the base of the tongue. A patient may be alarmed when looking at the tongue to notice these normal structures and mistake them for a serious disease. The foliate linguae on the margin of the tongue near the anterior pillar of the fauces may cause similar concern. The ***top arrow*** indicates the circumvallate papillae. The ***bottom arrow*** points to the foliate linguae.

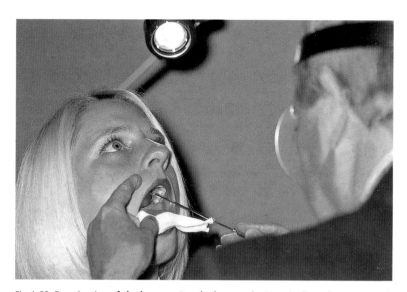

Fig. 1.60 Examination of the larynx using the laryngeal mirror (indirect laryngoscopy). A good view of the larynx is obtained with most patients. The valleculae, pyriform fossae, arytenoids, ventricular bands, and cords should all be clearly seen. It requires some inhibition of the gag reflex by the patient, and a local anesthetic lozenge or spray may be necessary. The tongue is held between the thumb and middle finger, and the upper lip retracted with the index finger. This examination is difficult in children, not only because they may be uncooperative, but because the *infantile epiglottis* is curved, unlike the "flat" adult epiglottis, and occludes a clear view of the larynx. Therefore, direct laryngoscopy under anesthetic may be necessary to diagnose the cause of hoarseness in a child. *Fiberoptic laryngoscopy* is necessary for seeing the larynx, which cannot be clearly seen on indirect laryngoscopy.

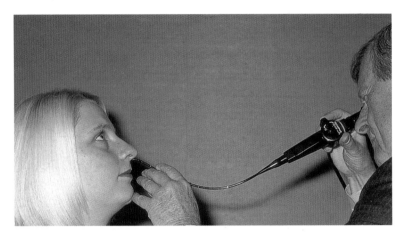

Fig. 1.**61 Fiberoptic endoscopy of the upper respiratory tract.** When the postnasal space and larynx are not clearly seen with routine mirror examination, the fiberoptic endoscope, which can be inserted through the nose, gives a view of the nasal fossae, postnasal space, and the larynx. A topical anesthetic is used on the nasal mucosa before the endoscopy is introduced. The field is small, however, and a TV camera may be attached to the endoscope so that a large view may be seen on the TV monitor—a view that may be shown to the patient.

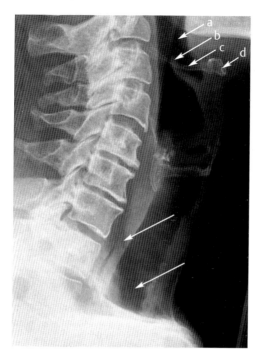

Fig. 1.**62 Lateral radiograph of the neck.** A lateral radiograph of the neck gives helpful information about the anatomy of the base of the tongue, larynx, trachea, and upper esophagus. The upper esophagus (upper arrow) is normally approximately the width of the trachea (lower arrow). An increase in the width of the esophagus is suggestive of significant pathology needing further investigation, such as a barium swallow radiograph or esophagoscopy. **a**, Base of tongue; **b**, epiglottis; **c**, glosso-epiglottic fold; **d**, hyoid bone.

Taste and Smell

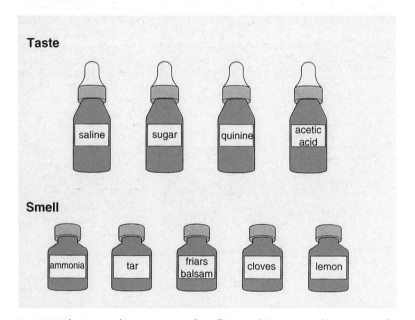

Fig. 1.**63 Solutions used to test taste and smell.** Four solutions are used to test taste. The solution is placed on one side of the tongue and the patient is asked to identify the taste: Sweet, salt, sour, or bitter. This is a relatively crude qualitative test. Testing for anosmia is done with a series of smell solutions for the patient to recognize.

No quantitative test for smell or taste is at present in routine clinical use. Anosmia is rarely the presenting symptom of a tumor in the nose or olfactory area (less than 1% of cases presenting with anosmia).

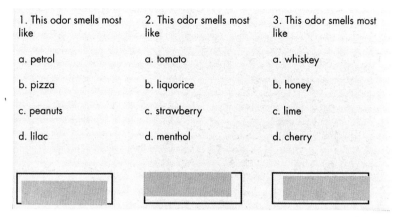

1. This odor smells most like	2. This odor smells most like	3. This odor smells most like
a. petrol	a. tomato	a. whiskey
b. pizza	b. liquorice	b. honey
c. peanuts	c. strawberry	c. lime
d. lilac	d. menthol	d. cherry

Fig. 1.**64 Anosmia "scratch card" tests:** A disk impregnated with a specific odor which is released when the disk is scratched with the fingernail. The smell identity is then marked on the card. Quantitative tests are not in routine clinical use, although "olfactometers" with measured odors for smell assessment are described.

Anosmia may be a complication of fracture of the anterior cranial fossa, or it may follow influenza; recovery is uncommon. Temporary anosmia will occur with severe nose obstruction. Anosmia is often linked with a complaint of impaired taste. This is usually found to be normal on testing.

The sensation of smell is an adjunct to the full subtle appreciation of taste. The dependence on smell for taste appreciation varies from person to person, so that a complaint of taste loss may or may not accompany anosmia.

One is dependent on the integrity of the patient's response to smell and taste tests. It is, therefore, often impossible to be certain in medicolegal cases whether anosmia or ageusia is genuine. With smell, a failure to identify a very strong stimulus such as ammonia suggests malingering, as cranial nerve V rather than I is involved.

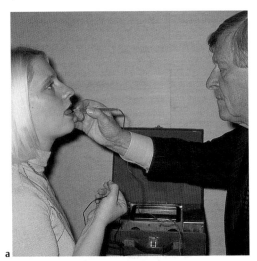

Fig. 1.65a, b Electrogustometry. Electricity has a metallic taste, and when a small current in µa is applied to the tongue, a quantitative reading can be obtained. The normal threshold on the margin of the tongue is between 5 and 30 µa. This more refined test of taste is also of interest in conditions such as facial palsy or acoustic neuroma, in which the chorda tympani nerve may be involved.

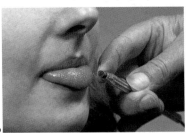

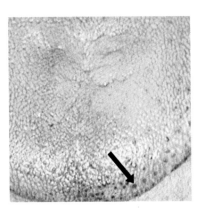

Fig. 1.66 The taste buds on the tongue are centered on the fungiform and circumvallate papillae. The *fungiform papillae* (arrowed) degenerate with age, and are prominent on a child's tongue. They also atrophy, as seen here, from the right side of the tongue to the mid-line, with the loss of the chorda tympani nerve, which may be divided in ear surgery. The filiform papillae account for the rough surface of the tongue and are not related to the taste sensation.

2 The Ear

The Pinna

Deformities

The pinna is formed from the coalescence of six tubercles, and development abnormalities are common.

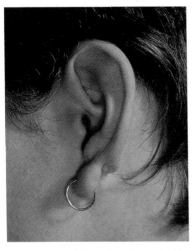

Fig. 2.**1 Minor deformities.** These are of little importance. This shows duplication of the lobule.

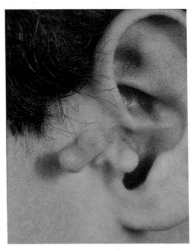

Fig. 2.**2 Hillocks (or accessory lobules).** These are commonly found anterior to the tragus, and are excised for cosmetic reasons. A small nodule of cartilage may be found underlying these hillocks. Hillocks, if treated soon after birth with a clip or ligature, necrose leaving no scar, avoiding later surgical excision.

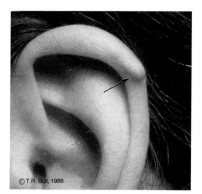

Fig. 2.**3 Darwin's tubercle (arrow).** A deformity of the pinna of phylogenetic interest. It is homologous to the tip of the mammalian ear and may be sufficiently prominent to justify surgical excision. Although Darwin's name is used for this tubercle, Woolmer gave the first description.

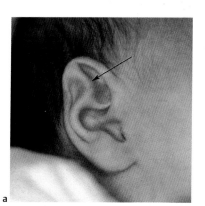

Fig. 2.**4a–c Stahl's bar** (arrow in **a**). This conspicuous congenital abnormality is treated with splints (**b**) used in the first 6–9 months of life (**a**, pre- and **c**, postsplinting). Also note small Darwin's tubercle (arrow in **c**). Surgical correction for Stahl's bar in later life is difficult, *so diagnosis soon after birth is important*.

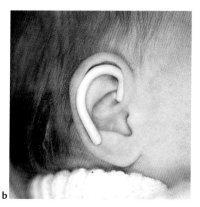

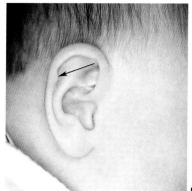

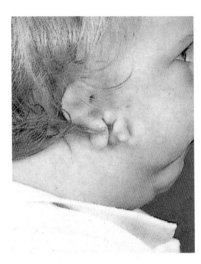

Fig. 2.**5 Microtia.** Absence of the pinna or gross deformity is often associated with meatal atresia and ossicular abnormalities. Faulty development of the 1st and 2nd branchial arches results in aural deformities which may be associated with hypoplasia of the maxilla and mandible, and eyelid deformities (Treacher-Collins syndrome, Fig. 2.**7b**). This type of pinna deformity is difficult to reconstruct.

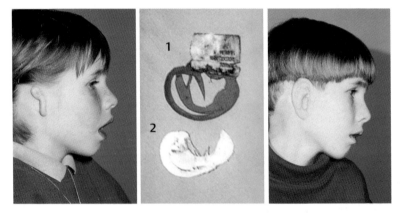

Fig. 2.**6 Surgical reconstruction for microtia.** Multiple surgical procedures are usually necessary, and a near-normal pinna is difficult to achieve. Rib cartilage grafts (1) are taken and fashioned (2) to act as a scaffold for local skin rotation flaps and free skin grafts. The reconstruction is a challenge for the innovative surgeon and results vary with the severity of pinna deformity.

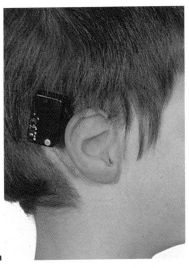
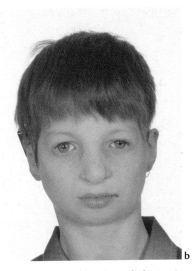

a   b

Fig. 2.7a, b Gross microtia with a bone-anchored prosthesis and hearing aid. If microtia is gross, a prosthesis rather than reconstruction is to be considered. Prosthetic ears have improved greatly in recent years. It is possible for these to be attached to the cranium using screws and plates (***osseo-integrated implants**,* see Fig. 1.**23**) with a bone-anchored hearing aid. This child with Treacher–Collins syndrome also has a healed tracheostomy site.

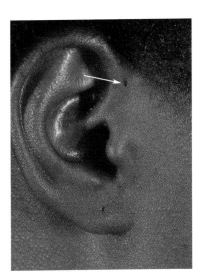

Fig. 2.8 Preauricular sinuses, which are closely related to the anterior crus of the helix, cause many problems. Discharge with recurrent swelling and inflammation may occur. The ***small opening of the sinus*** (arrow) ***is easily missed on examination***, particularly when it is concealed, as may rarely be the case, behind the fold of the helix, rather than in the more obvious anterior site.

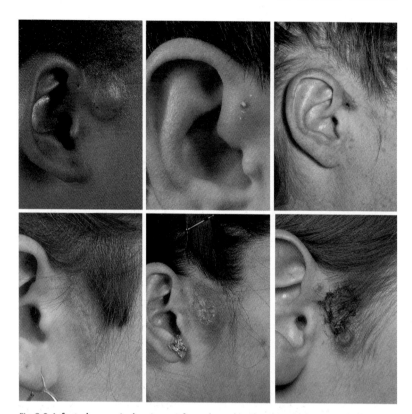

Fig. 2.9 **Infected preauricular sinus.** A furuncle or skin ulceration in this site is diagnostic of an underlying infected preauricular sinus. Quite extensive skin loss can occur in this site with recurrent infection of a preauricular sinus. The variation in the appearance of an infected preauricular sinus is striking, but the site in the preauricular region is diagnostic.

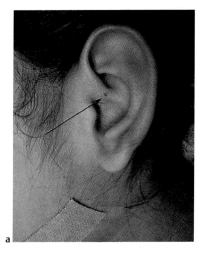

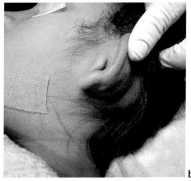

Fig. 2.**10 a Rare site of preauricular sinus.** The punctum is close to the root of the helix as seen here (arrow). **b** Infection causes displacement of the ear.

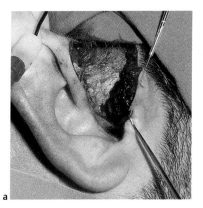

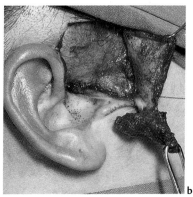

Fig. 2.**11 Preauricular sinus excision.** A furuncle or skin inflammation, which may be quite extensive in this preauricular site, is invariably related to a preauricular sinus. Careful examination for the sinus must be made. Excision when the infection is quiescent is necessary and this, although minor surgery, is not easy.

A long-branched and lobular structure must be excised. Incomplete excision of the tract leads to further infection and the need for revision surgery. To ensure complete excision of the preauricular sinus, the extension of an endaural incision as shown is needed, with reflection of the skin anteriorly down to the temporal facia. If the sac is injected with a dye it is better defined, and it is possible to be certain of complete excision. The sac is dissected from its deep aspect towards the sinus puncture, which is excised with an ellipse of skin.

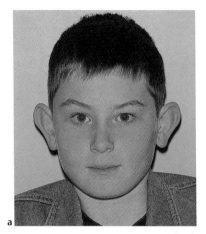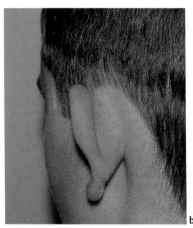

a   b

Fig. 2.**12 Prominent ears.** The fold of the antihelix is either absent or poorly formed in a prominent ear; it is not simply that the angle between the posterior surface of the conchal cartilage and the cranium is more "open." Parents and child may be offended by the diagnosis of "bat or lop" ears, although these terms are commonly used.

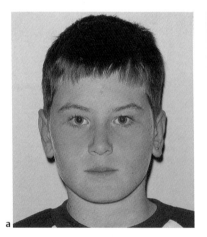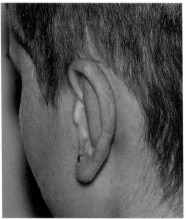

a   b

Fig. 2.**13 Surgical correction** aims to give a natural-looking ear. Techniques aim to avoid a "pinned back" appearance with a sharp, tender antihelix. Reshaping of the cartilage of the pinna is necessary, and recurrence follows simple excision of postauricular skin. Surgical correction of prominent ears is not straightforward and recurrence may occur. A prominent ear noted at birth (the deformity may develop in the few months after birth) can be cured with splinting (see p. 54), avoiding the need for later surgery.

Prominent ears are best corrected between the ages of four and six years at the beginning of school. There is, however, no additional surgical problem in correcting adult ears. Youngsters may be the subject of considerable ridicule in early years because of bat ears and, therefore, surgical correction is not to be deferred.

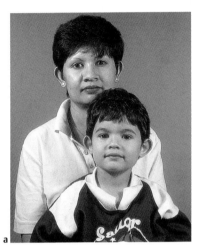 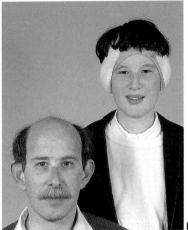

a   b

Fig. 2.**14 Bat ears** are often familial (**a**).
The son (**b**) has the firm ear dressing required for five to ten days after operation for prominent ears.

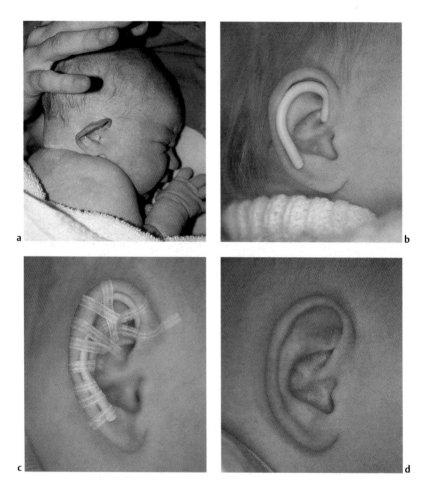

Fig. 2.**15a–d Prominent ears are often apparent either at or soon after birth.** In the first six months of life the elastic cartilage of the ear is "moldable." **a–d** demonstrate how a baby's ear can be molded to give a normal shape and produce an antihelix. After the age of one year, however, the cartilage spring is usually resistant to "molding" techniques.

Earrings

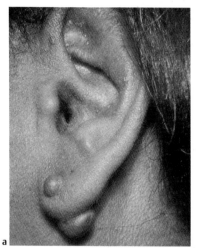

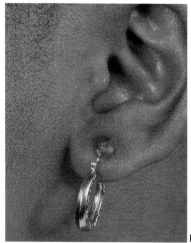

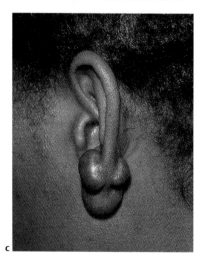

Fig.2.**16a–c Keloid formation** is common in black patients, and is difficult to treat.

Recurrence follows excision, and repeated excision may lead to huge keloid formation (**c**).

Radiotherapy or local triamcinolone injections following excision reduce the incidence of recurrence of the keloid. Pressure at the site of keloid excision has also been shown to reduce recurrence. Special pressure clip-on earrings are available to apply to the ear lobe after operation. Keloid formation is common near the ear and on the neck, *but is very rare in the middle third of the face*.

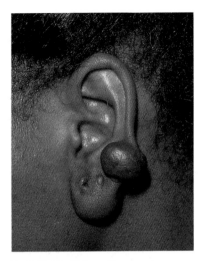

Fig. 2.**17 Keloid formation may be unpredictable:** a normal ear punctum from an earring puncture is adjacent to a large earring keloid.

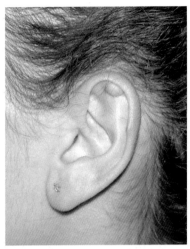

Fig. 2.**18 "High" ear piercing shows** the unpredictable nature of keloids. (No keloid at lobule earring site.)

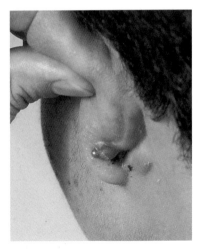

Fig. 2.**19 An infected granuloma** at the site of earring insertion.

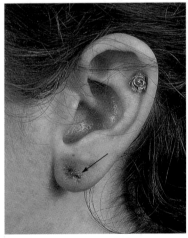

Fig. 2.**20 Nickel sensitivity** limits the use of certain earrings and has caused eczema on the lobule (arrow).

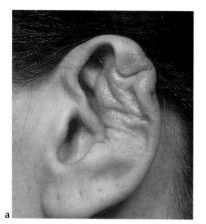

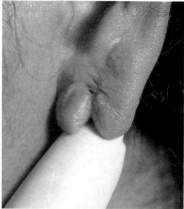

Fig. 2.**22 Trauma.** Traumatic "cutting-out" when the earring is pulled by a baby or adult in ill-humor. Infection at the time the sleepers are inserted is another hazard (see Fig. 2.**19**). Surgical repair requires a Z-plasty, for simple excision and suturing may cause "notching" of the lobule.

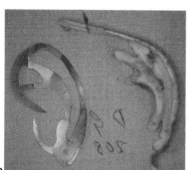

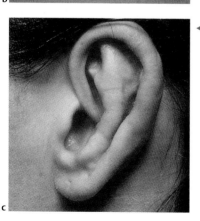

◄ Fig. 2.**21a–c "High" ear piercing** (Fig. 2.**20**, arrow) complicated by infection (frequently pseudomonas) may lead to abscess formulation. The puncture with high ear piercing (unlike the lobule) punctures cartilage and may lead to the additional problem of cartilage infection—perichondritis. Abscess incision with drainage, splinting, and antibiotic therapy (e.g., ciprofloxacin) is needed. Permanent deformity of the pinna may result, requiring a difficult plastic surgical repair (**a**). This involves taking a rib graft and modeling this to reconstruct the absent helix, antihelix, and scaphoid fossa of the pinna (**b; c,** post-op.).

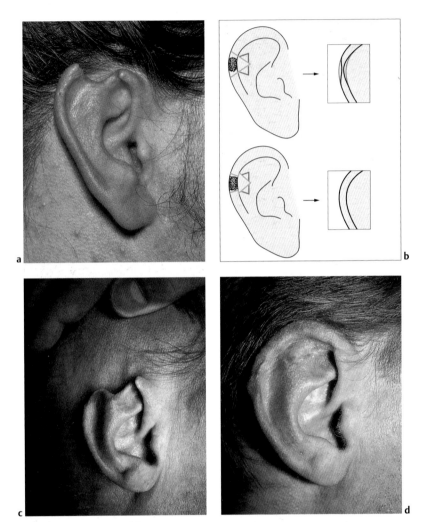

Fig. 2.**23a–d Trauma to the pinna.** The projecting and obvious pinna is a frequent site for trauma. Partial or complete avulsion is common. This loss of tissue is from a bite. Although small loss of the periphery of the helix can be closed with a wedge excision, larger loss (**c**) requires more complex surgical repair involving cartilage graft reconstruction of the helix (**d**).

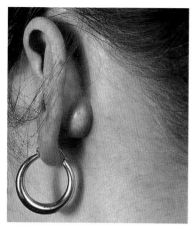

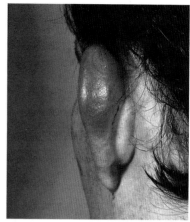

a

Fig. 2.**24 A sebaceous cyst** near the site of an earring puncture. The punctum is just apparent and is diagnostic. Sebaceous cysts are common behind the ear, particularly in the postaural sulcus.

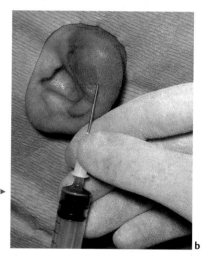

b

Fig. 2.**25a–c Hematomas of the pinna following trauma.** Bruising with minimal swelling settles (**a**). A hematoma or collection of serous fluid, however, is common, and these, particularly if recurrent from frequent injury and left untreated, will result in a **"cauliflower ear."** The fluid, if aspirated with a syringe (**b, c**), usually recurs, and incision and drainage may be necessary. Some thickening, however, of the underlying cartilage invariably takes place, and a return to a completely normal-shaped pinna is not usual. A spontaneous swelling of the pinna may present (a pseudocyst), also treated with incision, drainage, and curetting.

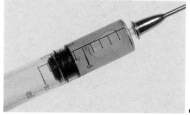

c

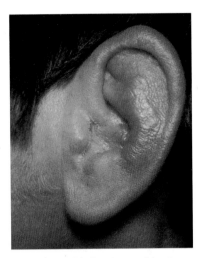

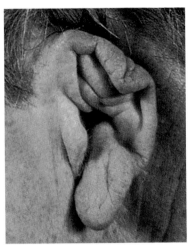

Fig. 2.**26 Perichondritis.** A painful red, tender, and swollen pinna accompanied by fever, following trauma or surgery, suggests an infection of the cartilage. The organism is frequently *Pseudomonas pyocyanea.*

Fig. 2.**27 Collapse of the pinna cartilage following perichondritis.** This happened prior to the availability of effective antibiotics. However, perichondritis is still a worrying complication which requires intensive antibiotic treatment. Collapsing or alteration of the shape of the pinna cartilage may also occur in relapsing polychondritis.

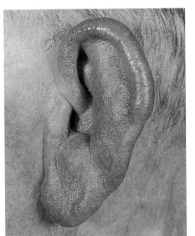

Fig. 2.**28 Relapsing polychondritis.** This is a rare inflammatory condition involving destruction and replacement with fibrous tissue of body cartilage. The elastic aural cartilage is replaced by fibrous tissue so that the ear has an unusual "felty" feel and does not have any "spring" on palpation.

The larynx cartilage also may be affected, causing hoarseness which may proceed to stridor. The nasal septum may collapse with a nasal saddle deformity (Figs. 3.**26a–d**). One or more of the lower limb joints are usually swollen and painful.

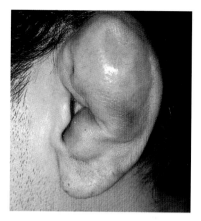

Fig. 2.**29a Pseudocyst.** This lesion which arises spontaneously and contains straw-coloured fluid on aspiration, is treated, to prevent deformity, in the same way as the swelling following trauma, i. e. helical rim incision, curetting, and compression dressing.

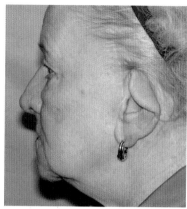

Fig. 2.**29b Relapsing polychondritis.** This inflammatory process may lead to cartilage destruction with loss of rigidity leading to pinna collapse.

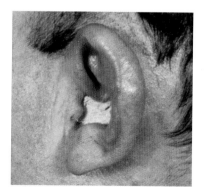

Fig. 2.**30 Iodoform sensitivity.** An antiseptic ear dressing commonly used contains bismuth, iodoform, and paraffin (B.I.P.). Sensitivity to iodoform may occur, and a red ear with marked irritation suggests this complication (rather than perichondritis, which is characterized by pain). ***Neomycin*** is one of the more commonly used topical antibiotics that may give rise to a skin sensitivity.

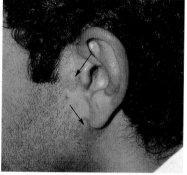

Fig. 2.**31 Burn scars** (arrows) in the ear region are evidence of the past use of cautery to relieve ear symptoms in childhood. In the Arab world, these burns are still common, and are known as ***chowes.***

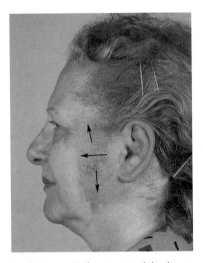

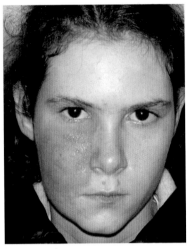

Fig. 2.**32a Erysipelas** is caused by hemolytic streptococci entering fissures in the skin near the orifice of the ear meatus (fissures such as those in otitis externa) and nose. A well-defined (arrows), raised erythema spreads to involve the face. This condition, which is often accompanied by malaise and fever, was serious in the preantibiotic era, but settles rapidly with penicillin.

Fig. 2.**32b** Erysipelas less commonly may follow infection from the nasal vestibule spreading to the facial skin.

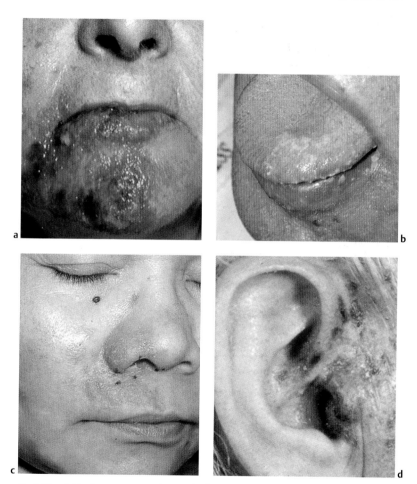

Fig. 2.33a–d The herpes zoster virus in the head and neck may affect the gasserian ganglion of cranial nerve V. Here the mandibular (**a**), with involvement of mucosa of the tongue (**b**), and the maxillary (**c**) divisions are involved. The vesicular type of skin eruption is confined to the distribution of the nerve. The ophthalmic division of V is most frequently involved, but all three divisions of V are rarely affected at the same time. The herpes zoster virus also involves the geniculate ganglion of cranial nerve VII (***Ramsay-Hunt syndrome or geniculate herpes***). Herpes affects the pinna and preauricular region (**d**), and is associated with a facial palsy. In most cases, there is also vertigo and sensorineural deafness. There is less likelihood of a full recovery of the facial palsy than in Bell's palsy (Fig. 2.**106**). Treatment is with antiviral agents, e. g., acyclovir, and oral steroids if not contraindicated.

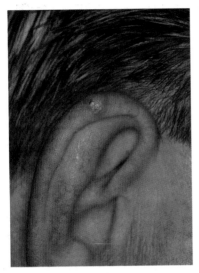

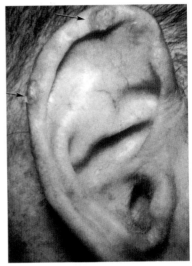

Fig. 2.**34 Basal cell carcinoma.** Ulcers on the helix are common. A long history suggests a basal cell carcinoma. This is treated with wedge resection. An ulcer of short duration suggests a squamous cell carcinoma or more rarely a melanoma, both of which require more extensive surgical resection.

Fig. 2.**35 Solar keratoses** (arrows). These warty growths affect the skin of the fair-headed when exposed to strong sunlight. They may become malignant. The skin of the helix may be affected with several of these keratoses.

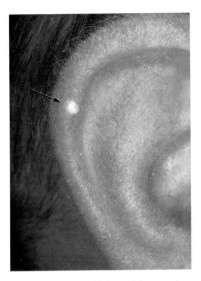

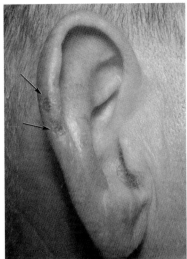

Fig. 2.**36 Gouty tophi** (arrow) from a characteristic lesion on the helix.

Fig. 2.**37 Inflammatory ulcers** (arrows) affect the helix and occasionally the antihelix. The lesions on the helix are blessed with a lengthy diagnosis—***chondrodermatitis nodularis helicis chronicis***—which presents as a longstanding intermittent ulceration.

It is primarily a chronic chondritis with secondary skin infection. A wedge resection of the ulcer and cartilage may be necessary, as the ulcer only heals temporarily with ointments.

Pressure on the ulcer, e. g., from a hard pillow, is a perpetuating factor. Relief of pressure with a soft "padding" dressing may lead to healing.

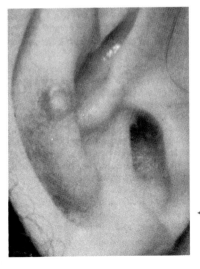

◄ Fig. 2.**38 Ulcers of the antihelix** are usually traumatic (on a particularly prominent antihelix fold). A basal or squamous cell carcinoma, however, may present on the antihelix.

The External Auditory Meatus

The skin of the external auditory meatus is migratory and does not desquamate.

Cleaning of the ear canal is therefore unnecessary—those who diligently clean their ears, or those of their children, with cotton buds, for example, hinder the migration of skin, predisposing to wax accumulation and otitis externa.

Some people have nonmigratory skin of the external auditory meatus and are susceptible to episodes of otitis externa. The meatus tends to become occluded with desquamated skin wax and debris, and periodic cleaning of the ear is necessary. The migration of meatal epithelium is also abnormal *in keratosis obturans. In this condition, desquamated epithelium accumulates and may form a large impacted mass in the meatus, causing erosion of the bony canal.*

In the past, skin grafts initially used for myringoplasty often failed or led to otitis externa, because skin taken from elsewhere on the body did not take on this migratory role. Fascia is used to graft the ear drum.

Although wax normally does not accumulate because of meatal skin migration, it may impact and cause a hearing loss, which may necessitate syringing, or suction clearance.

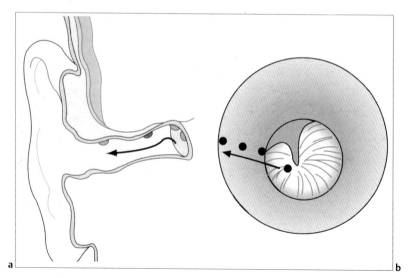

a

b

Fig. 2.**39a–f A migrating ink dot.**

Fig. 2.**39c–f** ▶

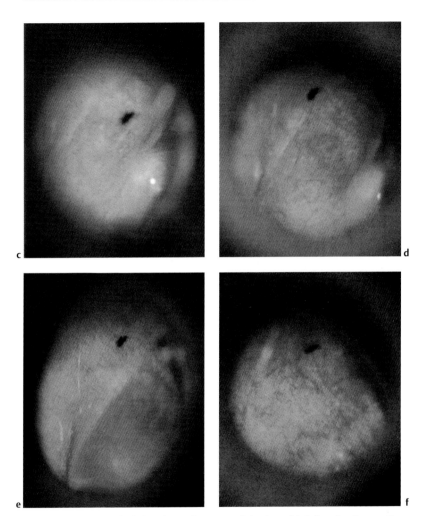

Fig. 2.**39c–f** A dot of ink, if placed near the center of the drum (**c**), is found to lie near the margin of the drum after three weeks (**d**), and between 6–12 weeks the dot migrates outwards on the meatal skin (**e, f**) to emerge in wax at the orifice of the meatus.

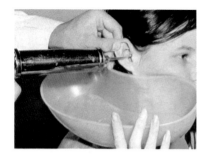

Fig. 2.**40 Syringing.** The rather large syringe of old-fashioned appearance has changed little in the past 100 years, and remains a simple and effective treatment for wax impaction. The pinna is pulled outwards and backwards to straighten the meatus, and water at body temperature is irrigated along the posterior wall of the ear. The water finds a passage past the wax, rebounds off the drum and pushes the wax outwards. Hard wax may require the use of softening oily drops before syringing.

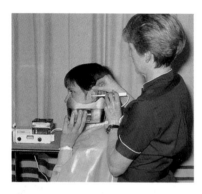

Fig. 2.**41   A modern ear syringe** with an electronically operated pump.

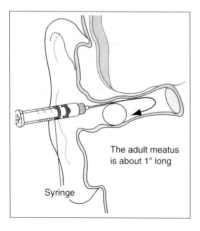

Fig. 2.**42 Syringing of the ear** requires expertise: undue force or clumsy technique may cause meatal skin damage with bleeding, a drum hematoma or perforation, and even sensorineural hearing loss.

A perforation, particularly in the presence of a thin drum, may be caused by over-penetration of the syringe nozzle. Care must also be taken to ensure that the nozzle is firmly connected to the syringe.

The adult meatus is about 1" long

Syringe

Syringing is not painful and pain means an error in technique, or that there is an otitis externa or perforation. Syringing an ear with a perforation may cause pain with vertigo and a subsequent otitis media with ear discharge.

Syringing may lead to an otitis externa and is to be avoided in those susceptible to this condition. ***An ear following stapedectomy or tympano-mastoid surgery should also not be syringed.***

Wax impaction in children is uncommon and it is not advisable to syringe the ears of a young child.

There are therefore occasions when suction clearance with the help of the microscope is necessary for the removal of ear wax.

Foreign Bodies

The main danger of a foreign body in the ear lies in its careless removal.

Syringing is effective and safe for small metallic foreign bodies. Vegetable foreign bodies, such as peas, swell with water and are better not syringed. Insects not uncommonly become impacted in the meatus, particularly in the tropics. Maggots cause a painful ear, and their removal is difficult. Insufflation of calomel powder is effective treatment.

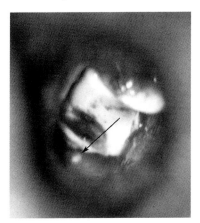

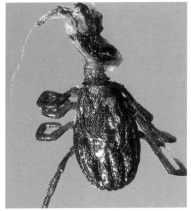

Fig. 2.**43 Foreign body in the ear.** An abrasion with bleeding is seen adjacent to the plastic foreign body. An arrow indicates the light reflex on the tympanic membrane beyond.

Fig. 2.**44 A tick foreign body in the ear.** The insect was adherent to the tympanic membrane, giving a sensation of discomfort and a deceptive drum appearance on examination; this insect was removed with syringing (a fragment of meatal skin is in the insect's mouth).

Previous attempts to remove a piece of plastic wedged in the child's meatus (Fig. 2.**43**) have led to bleeding in the meatus. The drum against which the foreign body impinges can be seen deep to the plastic.

One must not persevere in attempts to remove an aural foreign body, particularly in a child, as a perforation is easily caused. If immediate removal with a hook or syringe is not effective, the patient must be admitted for removal under general anesthetic with the help of the microscope. It is often dangerous to use forceps to remove an aural foreign body, since the object easily slips from the jaws of the forceps to go deeper into the meatus.

Otitis Externa

Eczema of the meatus and pinna (see Fig. 2.**45**) may be associated with eczema elsewhere, particularly in the scalp, or it may be an isolated condition affecting only one ear. Itching is the main symptom, with scanty discharge. The eczematous type of otitis externa usually settles with the use of a topical corticosteroid and antibiotic drop. The use of Quinolone antibiotics may be favored as there will be no theoretical risk of inner ear toxicity. Cleaning of the meatus may also be necessary, either with cotton wool on a probe, or suction and the Zeiss microscope. Otitis externa tends to recur.

The patient should avoid over-diligent cleaning of the meatus, or scratching the ear with the finger, probes, or cotton wool buds. Cotton wool buds, if used, should only be used to the orifice of the meatus. Water entering the ear during washing or swimming also predisposes to the recurrence of otitis externa.

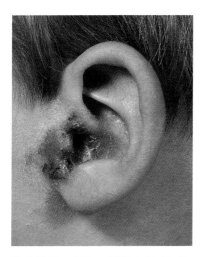

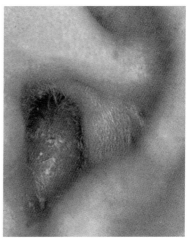

Fig. 2.**45 Eczematous otitis externa.** Eardrop sensitivity may worsen an otitis externa. Chloramphenicol drops caused this condition. Neomycin less commonly causes similar reactions. *Patients should be advised to discontinue eardrops that cause an increase in irritation or that are painful.*

Fig. 2.**46 A furuncle** in the meatus is the other common type of otitis externa. It is characterized by pain; pain on movement of the pinna or on inserting the auriscope is diagnostic of a furuncle. *Diabetes mellitus* must be excluded with recurrent furuncles.

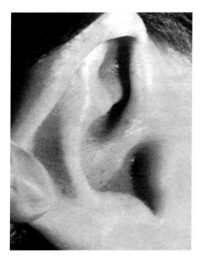

Fig. 2.**47 Furunculosis.** This is a generalized infection of the meatal skin. Pain is severe and the canal is narrowed or occluded so that examination with the auriscope is extremely painful and no view of the deep meatus is possible. A swab of the pus should be taken, and treatment is with systemic antibiotics, e.g. Ciprofloxacin, and a meatal dressing (e.g., glycerine and ichthyol, or a corticosteroid cream with an antibiotic).

The organism may be transferred by the patient's finger from the nasal vestibules, and a nasal swab is a relevant investigation, particularly with recurrent furuncles. The lymph nodes adjacent to the pinna are enlarged with a furuncle or furunculosis, and a tender mastoid node may mimic a cortical mastoid abscess.

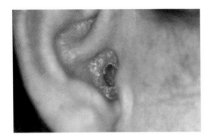

Fig. 2.**48 Chronic otitis externa** persisting for years may eventually lead to meatal stenosis and rarely to closure of the ear canal.

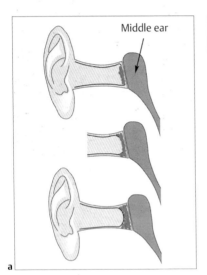

Middle ear

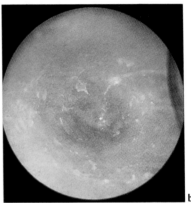

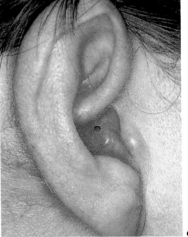

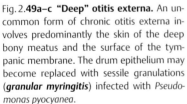

Fig. 2.**49a–c "Deep" otitis externa.** An uncommon form of chronic otitis externa involves predominantly the skin of the deep bony meatus and the surface of the tympanic membrane. The drum epithelium may become replaced with sessile granulations (**granular myringitis**) infected with *Pseudomonas pyocyanea*.

In protracted cases of this type of otitis externa, the skin of the deep meatus and drum becomes thickened and "funneled" with meatal atresia. The resulting conductive hearing loss is extremely difficult to treat surgically once this condition is quiescent.

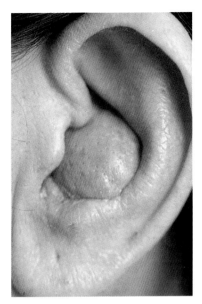

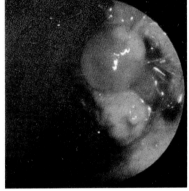

Fig.2.**50 Kimura's disease.** A rare, benign inflammatory condition more common in Asians and often affecting the head and neck. The condition was first described by T. Kimura, a Japanese physician, in 1948. Surgical excision for cosmesis and histology to confirm the diagnosis. The differential diagnoses include angiolymphoid hyperplasia, Kaposi sarcoma, and pyogenic granuloma. It may be mistaken for serious pathology.

Fig.2.**51 "Malignant" otitis externa** is a rare and serious form of otitis externa to which elderly diabetics are particularly susceptible. Granulation tissue is found in the meatus infected with *Pseudomonas* and anaerobic organisms. This granulation tissue tends to erode deeply, involving the middle and inner ear, the bone of the skull base with extension to the brain, and also the great vessels of the neck. If uncontrolled, the condition may be fatal.

Intense antibiotic therapy sometimes associated with surgical drainage of the affected areas is necessary. It is not a "malignant" condition in the histological sense, for the biopsies of granulation tissue show inflammatory changes only. "Necrotizing" otitis externa may be more accurate, but "malignant" indicates the serious clinical nature.

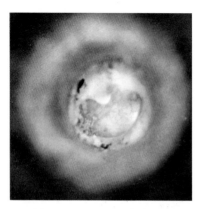

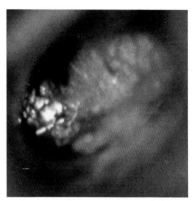

Fig. 2.**52 Otitis externa secondary to discharge via a drum perforation** is initially treated (an ear swab having been taken for culture and sensitivity) with cleaning of the meatus and the instillation of the appropriate antibiotic and corticosteroid drops. If the condition persists with marked irritation and pain, a ***fungal otitis externa*** should be suspected. In persistent infection, the meatus contains a cocktail of drops, pus, and desquamated skin. In fungal infections, as shown here, the dark spores of *Aspergillus niger* and white mycelium of *Candida albicans* can be seen. Thorough cleaning of the meatus precedes treatment with a topical antifungal agent.

The meatal skin infection is introduced from outside—usually from the patient's finger, or from water, particularly after swimming.

The infection, however, may be from the middle ear if there is a perforation, and discharge from chronic otitis media may be the cause of a persistent otitis externa. Otitis externa rarely damages the tympanic membrane. With fungal otitis externa, however, and the presence of a granular myringitis, a perforation may ensue.

Fig. 2.**53 Bullous otitis externa (bullous myringitis).** This unusual otitis externa frequently follows influenza or an upper respiratory tract infection. A complaint of earache followed by bleeding, then followed by relief of pain is diagnostic of this condition.

Examination shows hemorrhagic blebs on the drum and meatus, similar to the vesicular eruption of herpes. If there is pyrexia with a conductive hearing loss, the otitis externa is associated with an otitis media, and systemic antibiotics are necessary. In the absence of pyrexia and hearing loss, this condition settles spontaneously without treatment.

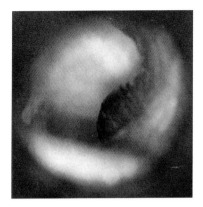

Fig. 2.54 Otitis externa with herpes zoster. Otitis externa occurs with herpes zoster (see Fig. 2.**33d**) involving either the gasserian or geniculate ganglion, and the vesicles may be hemorrhagic.

Carcinomas and melanomas in the skin of the external auditory meatus are rare, but any persistent granulation or skin lesion should be biopsied.

Osteomas

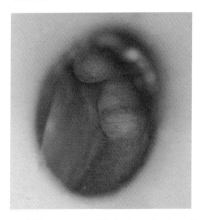
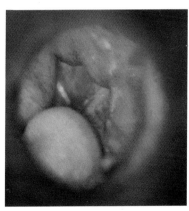

Fig. 2.55 Osteomas. White, bony, hard swellings in the deep meatus are a common finding during routine examination. They usually remain small and symptom free, and tend to be symmetrical in both ears.

Swimmers are susceptible to these lesions, which are sometimes called *"swimmer's osteomas."* There is experimental evidence to show that irrigation of the bony meatus with cold water produces a periostitis that leads to osteoma formation. Histologically, these bony lesions are hyperostosis, rather than a bony tumor, so that the term "osteoma," although established, is not strictly correct.

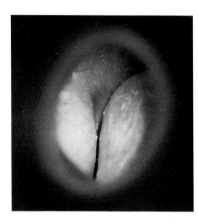

Fig. 2.**56 Large osteomas** may narrow the meatus to a chink so that wax accumulates and is difficult to syringe. Otitis externa is also a complication.

These osteomas, therefore, may require surgical removal with a microdrill. They should not be removed with a gouge, for a fracture with bleeding in the remaining osteoma is a probable complication, causing damage to the facial nerve and resulting in facial palsy.

It is rare for osteomas to occlude the meatus completely, and in almost all cases no treatment is required.

The Tympanic Membrane and Middle Ear

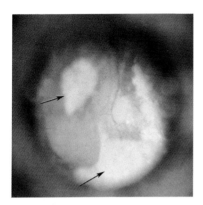

Fig. 2.**57 "Chalk" patches.** White areas of *tympanosclerosis* (arrows) are common findings on examination of the drum. They are of little significance in themselves, and the hearing is often normal. A past history of otorrhea in childhood or grommet insertion is usual. Chalk patches do occur with no apparent past otitis media.

Extensive tympanosclerosis with a rigid drum is a sequela of past otitis media, and the ossicles, too, may be fixed or noncontinuous.

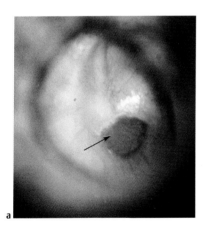

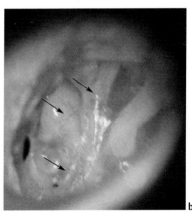

a   b

Fig. 2.**58a, b Scarring of the drum. a** A gossamer-thin membrane can be seen to close this previously well-defined central perforation (arrow). At first sight with the auriscope, a central perforation would appear to be the diagnosis; more careful examination with a pneumatic otoscope will show that this thin membrane moves and seals the defect, giving reassurance that the drum is intact.

b *Scarring of the drum with retraction* onto the round window, promontory, and incus (arrows) is also evidence of past otitis media. It is sometimes difficult to be sure whether this type of drum is intact; a thin layer of epithelium indrawn onto the middle-ear structures may seal the middle ear, and examination with the operating microscope may be necessary to be certain of an intact drum.

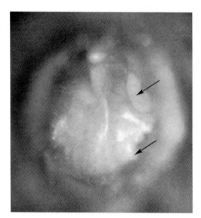

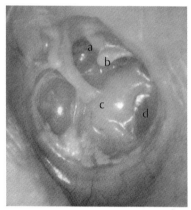

Fig. 2.**59 Scarred tympanic membrane.** A scarred tympanic membrane in which the drum has become atelectatic and indrawn onto the long process of the incus and promontory (arrows).

Fig. 2.**60 A retracted tympanic membrane** which is thin and indrawn onto the long process of the incus (**a**), head of the stapes (**b**), promontary (**c**), and round window (**d**). The stapedius tendon is also seen in this panoramic view obtained with a fiberoptic endoscope.

Perforations

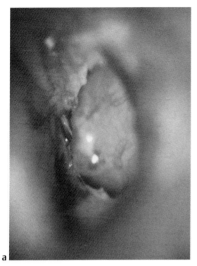

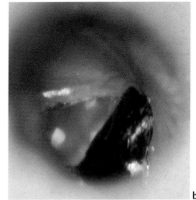

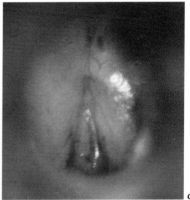

Fig. 2.**61a–c Traumatic perforation.** A blow on the ear with the hand is a common cause of traumatic perforation which has an ***irregular margin*** (**a**), and there is fresh blood or a blood clot (**b**) on the drum.

The defect is frequently slit-shaped (**c**). Pain and transient vertigo at the time of injury are followed by a tinnitus and hearing loss.

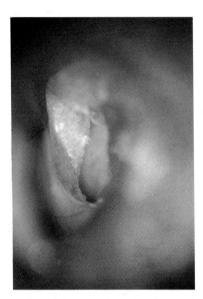

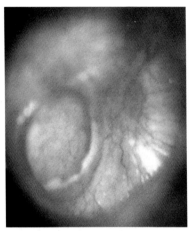

Fig. 2.**62 Healing perforation.** *Almost all traumatic perforations heal spontaneously* within two months, a thin membrane growing across the defect. Traumatic perforations are usually central, but if the perforation extends to the annulus, healing may not occur. The extremely large traumatic perforations may also fail to close spontaneously.

Taking care to avoid water entering the middle ear and avoiding inflating the middle ear with the Valsalva maneuver are the only precautions the patient need take.

A middle-ear infection with discharge is the commonest complication, usually settling with a course of topical and systemic antibiotics. Blast injuries, barotrauma, foreign bodies or their careless removal, and even over-enthusiastic kissing of the ear may also cause traumatic perforations.

Fig. 2.**63 Central perforation.** Acute otitis media with pus under pressure in the middle ear may rupture the drum, and although healing usually occurs, a permanent perforation can result. These perforations are usually central. A small perforation may be symptom-free, but episodes of otorrhea with head colds and after swimming are common, along with a conductive hearing loss.

The otorrhea tends to be profuse and mucopurulent, and may be intermittent or persistent. This type of central perforation, when dry, is successfully closed with a fascial graft (**myringoplasty**).

Other complications with central perforations are rare, so they are described as **"safe" perforations**. A central perforation may persist after an episode of acute otitis media and otorrhea in childhood. Myringoplasty is usually delayed in children since closure by puberty is common. If, however, the upper respiratory tract is free of infection, and the perforation is the site of recurrent infections with impaired hearing, these are indications to proceed with myringoplasty in childhood.

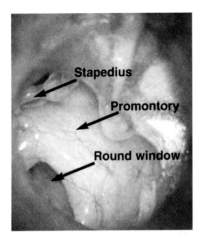

Fig. 2.**64 Marginal perforation.** A perforation may reach the annulus posteriorly and is called marginal. The middle-ear structures are frequently seen through the perforation.

The well-defined margin of the round window is particularly obvious, and the promontory, incudostapedial joint, and stapedius are also apparent.

Fig. 2.**65 A posterior marginal perforation of the eardrum,** taken with the fiberoptic camera, showing the round window and head of the stapes. A thin fibrous connection can be seen (arrow) which connects to the necrotic long process of the incus. This type of ossicular discontinuity is a common cause of conductive hearing loss following otitis media (with or without a perforation). Ossicular reconstruction surgery will restore the hearing.

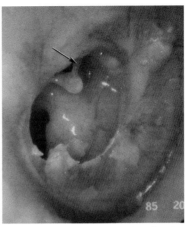

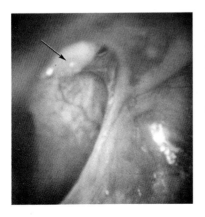

Fig. 2.**66 Squamous epithelium on the incus.** The marginal perforation may enable squamous epithelium to migrate into the middle ear. In this ear, white squamous epithelium has formed on the incus (arrow). Marginal perforations, therefore, are described as "unsafe" since there is a ***risk of cholesteatoma*** (see Fig. 2.**68**).

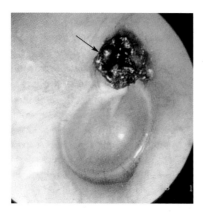

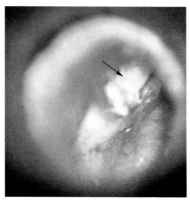

Fig. 2.**67 Attic perforation.** Debris adherent to the pars flaccida of the drum (arrow) suggests an underlying attic perforation. ***Perforations of the pars flaccida*** (attic perforations) are invariably associated with ***cholesteatoma*** formation.

Fig. 2.**68 Cholesteatoma.** The debris, when removed, exposes a white mass of epithelium characteristic of a cholesteatoma (arrow). Cholesteatoma is not a neoplasm; it is simply squamous epithelium in the middle ear.

If ignored, it increases in size, becomes infected, and is associated with a scanty, fetid otorrhea. It may erode bone, leading to serious complications. Extension to involve the dura with intracranial infection may occur, and the facial nerve and labyrinth too may be eroded. The extent of the cholesteatoma determines the danger: A small attic pocket of epithelium is relatively harmless, and can be removed with suction, but an extensive mass of epithelium is dangerous and needs exploration and removal via a mastoidectomy approach.

A chronic discharging ear is not painful, and persistent pain and headache, or severe vertigo, strongly suggest an intracranial complication or labyrinth.

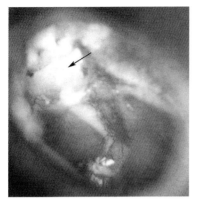

Fig. 2.**69 Cholesteatoma.**

Cholesteatoma erodes the bony wall of the deep meatus so that a pocket containing white debris forms in the posterior–superior aspect of the drum (arrow).

The complete etiology of the cholesteatoma is not understood. Migration of epithelium into the middle ear via an attic or posterior marginal perforation certainly accounts for most cholesteatomas. However, cholesteatoma may occur behind an intact drum, and may form with central perforations. Eustachian tube dysfunction with a negative pressure in the middle ear, if longstanding, leads to a chronic middle-ear effusion (chronic otitis media with effusion) and a retracted drum. The pars flaccida retracts and may give the opportunity for a pocket of cholesteatoma to develop. In this picture of cholesteatoma, the remainder of the drum is a golden color and fluid is present in the middle ear. This longstanding effusion may have been responsible for this cholesteotoma formation.

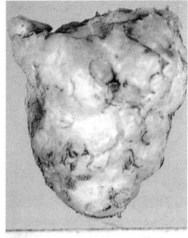

1 | **2**

Fig. 2.**70 A cholesteatoma** of 2 cm diameter removed at mastoidectomy presents the typical well-defined mass of white epithelium. The bone erosion that this mass causes shows on mastoid radiographs and computed tomography (CT) or magnetic resonance imaging (MRI) scans.

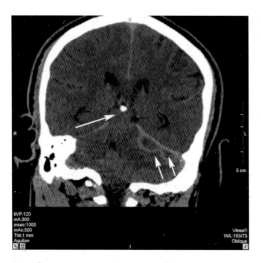

Fig. 2.**71 Serious complications** may arise from spread of infection from chronic suppurative otitis media (CSOM) with or without cholesteatoma, but are uncommon. Labyrinthitis, facial nerve damage, and intracranial infection may all occur. The figure shows posterior fossa brain abscesses (lower arrows) (a ventriculoperitoneal shunt is in place; upper arrow).

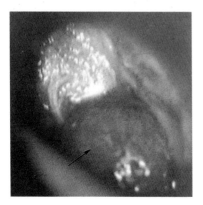

Fig. 2.**72 Aural granulation.** *In the same way that epithelium may migrate through a perforation into the middle ear, mucous membrane may extrude outwards to the meatus.* Middle-ear mucous membrane extruding through a perforation (arrow) becomes infected and presents with a discharging ear. An aural granulation is seen in the deep meatus. Granulation may also form on the drum of the margin of the perforation, and rarely granulation tissue forms on an intact drum in otitis externa (granular myringitis) (see Fig. 2.**49**).

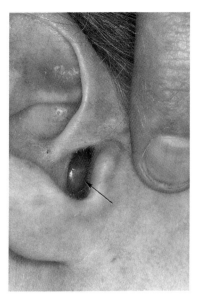

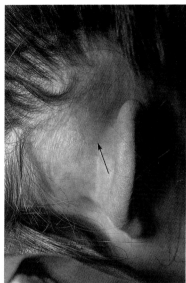

Fig. 2.**73 Aural polyp.** If the growth of granulation tissue is exuberant, a pedunculated polyp develops, which may present at the orifice of the meatus (arrow). Granulations and polyps commonly arise from the tympanic annulus posteriorly, but the originating site may also be the mucous membrane of the promontory, eustachian tube orifice, and antrum and aditus. Careful and thorough removal of polyps and granulation tissue to their site of origin is necessary. If the polyp is associated with cholesteatoma, removal by mastoid approach is required.

Fig. 2.**74 Mastoid abscess.** A red, acutely tender swelling filling the postauricular sulcus (arrow), and pushing the pinna conspicuously forwards and outwards, is characteristic of a mastoid abscess.

In the past, mastoidectomy was needed for an acute mastoid abscess complicating acute otitis media. This was extremely common in the preantibiotic era, and required exenteration of the mastoid air cells (**cortical mastoidectomy**). The operation is now rarely performed in countries where antibiotics are available.

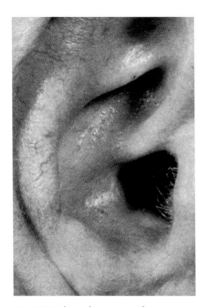

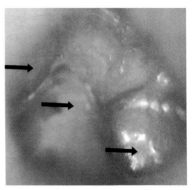

Fig. 2.**76 Auriscope view.** With the auriscope, a ridge (containing the facial nerve) can be seen separating the drum anteriorly from the epithelized cavity posteriorly. Failure of the mastoid cavity to epithelize results in an infected cavity with discharge.

(Top arrow: mastoid cavity; middle arrow: facial ridge with the bone overlying the descending portion of the facial nerve; bottom arrow: tympanic membrane.)

Fig. 2.**75 Enlarged meatus after mastoidectomy.** A more extensive type of mastoidectomy is, however, still necessary for cholesteatoma which has extended beyond the middle ear. This operation often alters the anatomy of the ear. Examination after operation will show an enlarged meatus. At operation the meatus is enlarged with a meatoplasty to allow access to the mastoid cavity, so that wax can be removed with a Jobson–Horne probe or with suction. This is usually necessary once or twice a year, as the skin of the mastoid cavity does not migrate satisfactorily and therefore wax accumulates. Water entering in the ear following mastoidectomy should be avoided; infection and otorrhea tend to follow. ***Syringing of a mastoid cavity is also to be avoided***, not only because of the possibility of subsequent otorrhea but because irrigation of water over the exposed lateral semicircular canal causes vertigo.

Surgical techniques aim to remove cholesteatoma without exteriorizing the mastoid cavity, so that relatively normal anatomy is maintained postoperatively, and hearing is maintained or improved (***intact canal wall tympanoplasty***), although this operation is not suitable for every case. Although avoiding a mastoid cavity, the intact canal wall tympanoplasty technique tends to conceal a recurrence of cholesteatoma. There are also surgical techniques to obliterate the mastoid cavity with muscle, fascia, or bone grafts.

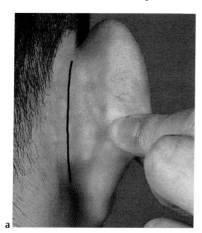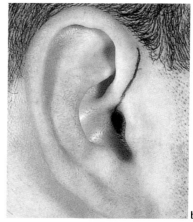

a   b

Fig. 2.**77a, b Postaural and endaural incisions.** These are two commonly used incisors for access to the middle ear and mastoid. The postaural incision (**a**) is preferred if extensive mastoid exenteration is planned. The incision lines are delineated here, but in these sites the scars are imperceptible.

Otitis Media

Otitis Media with Effusion (so-called "Glue ear" in Children)

A middle-ear effusion is a common cause of conductive hearing loss. It may occur when either a head cold or barotrauma interferes with eustachian tube function, and it often follows acute otitis media. ***A postnasal space neoplasm*** may also cause eustachian tube dysfunction, and is to be excluded in any adult with a ***persistent otitis media with effusion.***

In children, otitis media with effusion is very common when adenoid tissue interferes with the eustachian tube. The middle-ear fluid tends to be tenacious (***"glue ear"***), unlike the thin, straw-colored exudate of adults.

The appearance of the drum is altered and the mobility reduced.

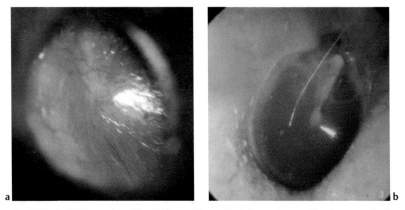

Fig. 2.**78a, b Otitis media with effusion with minimal drum change.** The drum may look only slightly different, with a brown color and some hyperemia. A confident diagnosis of middle-ear fluid can only be made if reduced mobility is demonstrated and impedance audiometry (Figs. **1.30**, 1.**31**) is needed for confirmation.

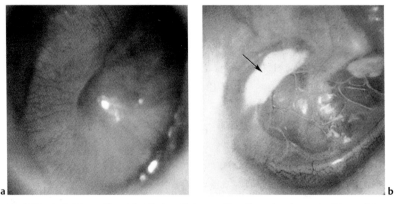

Fig. 2.**79a, b Otitis media with effusion ("glue ear"). a** The color change in this condition is often diagnostic, as well as the reduced mobility. The golden-brown color showing through the translucent drum is readily apparent in the inferior part of the tympanic membrane.

  b A photograph with a fiberoptic camera gives a panoramic view of the deep meatus and membrane. Bubbles within the fluid and levels appearing as a hairline in the drum may be seen. A "chalk" patch is also seen (arrow).

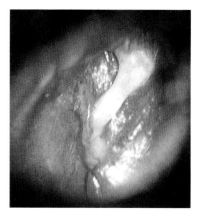 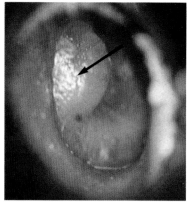

Fig. 2.**80 Otitis media with effusion with marked drum change.** The change is frequently gross, making the diagnosis obvious, with a golden color, a retracted membrane, and a prominent malleus.

Fig. 2.**81 A vesicle on the drum** (arrow) often occurs in children's glue ear.

The full etiology of the eustachian tube dysfunction causing otitis media with effusion is at present unknown. Opinions, therefore, differ on the treatment, particularly that of children's "glue ears." Adenoid tissue in the region of the eustachian tube orifice predisposes to "glue ears," and adenoid removal is frequently necessary.

Glue Ear

"Glue ear" is common between the ages of three and six years, and uncommonly persists after 11 years. The hearing loss is often slight and varies with colds. The self-limiting nature of the condition calls for conservative treatment, but "glue ears" are not to be ignored.

A marked and persistent hearing loss, interfering with schooling, necessitates surgery. Episodes of transient otalgia are common with "glue ears," and frequent attacks of acute otitis media may occur. The drum may also become retracted and flaccid with prolonged middle-ear fluid. These features may necessitate insertion of a grommet to reventilate the middle ear.

With glue ear associated with upper respiratory tract symptoms or with proven atopy, the use of an antihistamine and nasal steroid spray assist the resolution of the middle-ear effusion.

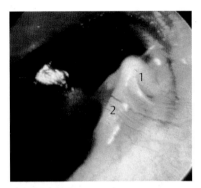

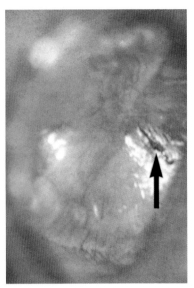

Fig. 2.**82 Blue drum.** The middle-ear effusion alters in composition, and at some stages in otitis media with effusion the drum appears blue in color—the so-called *"blue drum."*

A similarly blue appearance of the tympanic membrane is seen following injury when bleeding occurs in the middle ear (hemotympanum). The conductive hearing loss associated with this injury resolves with resorption of the middle-ear hematoma. A persisting conductive hearing loss following injury, however, suggests injury to the ossicles with an ossicular discontinuity (see Fig. 2.**94**).

Otitis media with effusion often settles spontaneously.

1, Lateral process of malleus; 2, handle of malleus.

Fig. 2.**83 Myringotomy.** If otitis media with effusion with poor hearing persists for over three months, myringotomy (under general anesthetic in children) with aspiration of the fluid is often necessary.

An arrow indicates the radial incision of the myringotomy into which the grommet may be inserted. The posterior/superior quadrant of the drum is not used to avoid injury to the underlying incus and stapes.

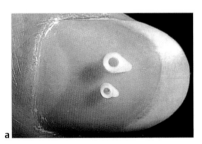

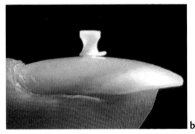

Fig. 2.**84a, b Grommets. a** The insertion of a grommet, a flanged Teflon tube, is frequently needed to avoid a recurrence of middle-ear fluid. **b** A mini-grommet causes less drum trauma, but extrusion is more rapid.

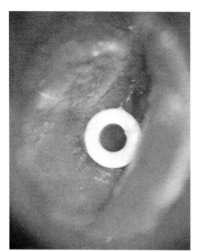

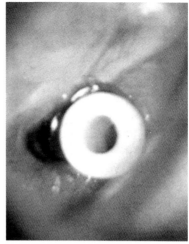

Fig. 2.85 Grommet insertion. A myringotomy incision in the posterior half of the drum may damage the incudostapedial joint or round window, and a grommet inserted posteriorly may cause incus necrosis from pressure on the long process: *An anterior or inferior radial myringotomy is a safer incision.*

Fig. 2.86 A grommet in place. The grommet tube ventilates the middle ear and acts instead of the eustachian tube. Hearing and the appearance of the drum both return to normal.

The grommet usually extrudes spontaneously between 6 and 18 months to leave an intact drum, and is found in wax in the meatus. With recurrent middle-ear fluid, repeated grommet insertion may be needed. If normal eustachian tube function has not returned and otitis media with effusion recurs, the grommet is replaced.

Tympanosclerosis and drum scarring ensue. This complication is also seen in untreated "glue ear." Minimal surgical trauma during grommet insertion is advisable. However, with a narrow ear canal, grommet insertion is not always technically easy.

The Patulous, or "Over-patent" Eustachian Tube

Obstruction of the eustachian tube is a common and frequently diagnosed disorder. Abnormal patency of the tube *(the patulous eustachian tube), however, is also not uncommon, and the diagnosis is frequently missed.*

The condition tends to occur in people who have lost weight or women who are taking "the pill" or are pregnant. The symptoms are of a sensation of blockage in the ear, with normal hearing or minimal loss. Patients may comment that they hear themselves breathe and eat, and hear their own voice "echo" in their ear. This sensation may alter with head movement (wrongly suggesting middle-ear fluid), and often is absent on lying down. Fortunately, the symptoms are usually minor and settle spontaneously. Reassurance and explanation suffice as treatment in most cases. Failure to make the diagnosis, however, and treatment of the condition as eustachian tube obstruction is common.

Chronic Otitis Media with Effusion

Middle-ear fluid, if persistent, may cause permanent changes in the drum. An otitis media with effusion can cause hearing loss for decades, and the diagnosis is frequently overlooked in a long-standing hearing loss. Impedance audiometry helps in diagnosis.

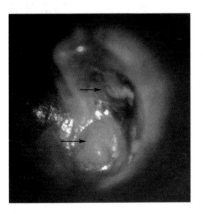

Fig. 2.**87 Grossly altered drum.** A brown color, with retraction of a flaccid membrane onto the ossicles and promontory, is seen with long-standing middle-ear fluid. (Bottom arrow: indrawn drum onto the promontory; top arrow: incudostapedial joint.)

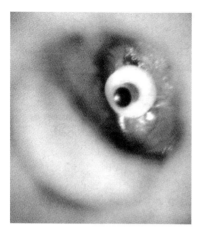

Fig. 2.88 Grommet occluded with exudate. Insertion of a grommet in these chronic adult cases may restore hearing, but frequently either the lumen of the grommet becomes occluded with exudate, which may extrude through the tube into the meatus, or a constant otorrhea occurs.

There is no successful treatment at present for chronic otitis media with effusion when this fails to respond to insertion of a grommet. A further problem with chronic otitis media with effusion is the return of middle-ear fluid with hearing loss when the grommet extrudes. A larger flanged grommet (long-term grommet) which remains in position longer, and periodic replacement are the present remedies.

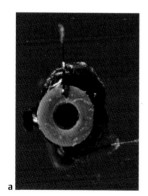

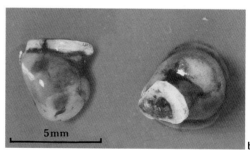

a

b

Fig. 2.**89 a The grommet lumen may also become obstructed with blood** if the myringotomy incision bleeds excessively. **b Infection with a granuloma may also occlude the lumen.** Granulomata arise as a result of biofilm formation. These complex bacterial aggregates appear to confer a degree of resistance to drug therapy. It is frequently necessary for the grommet to be removed.

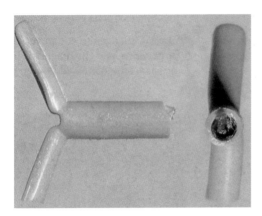

Fig. 2.**90   Occlusion of the grommet lumen.** Excess bleeding at the time of insertion may cause this problem, or subsequent occlusion with serous exudate. There are various designs of grommet or ventilation tube, and this Y-shaped tube shows the narrow lumen to be occluded.

Acute Otitis Media

Earache with conductive hearing loss and fever accompanying a head cold characterize acute otitis media. The drum is red and the landmarks are obscured; drum distension and pulsation may be seen.

Otitis media is common in children, probably due to their short, wide eustachian tube and the presence of adenoids which may be infected near the orifice. Rupture of the tympanic membrane in acute otitis media is not uncommon and muco-purulent otorrhea ensues with a pulsatile discharge. Penicillin is invariably curative, and complications are rare.

The middle-ear infection frequently settles without otorrhea, but if the drum does rupture, a pulsating muco-purulent discharge filling the meatus is diagnostic of otitis media. A swab for culture and sensitivity is taken in these cases, although the ear usually becomes dry within 48 hours of penicillin therapy, and the perforation closes in most cases with little or no scarring.

Acute mastoiditis, previously serious and common, is almost unheard of where antibiotics are available. Myringotomy and cortical mastoidectomy are operations of the past for acute otitis media.

Otitis media with effusion after the acute attack is the main complication today.

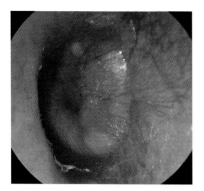

Fig. 2.**91 Acute otitis media** with bulging and hyperemia of the posterior-superior quadrant of the tympanic membrane. This is the typical early appearance of acute otitis media photographed with a fiberoptic camera.

Glomus Tumor

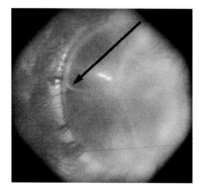

Fig. 2.**92 Glomus jugulare tumor.** A photograph, via the fiberoptic endoscope, showing a glomus jugulare tumor presenting, as is characteristic, with a hyperemia in the lower half of the drum. Middle-ear fluid is often present, and a meniscus is also seen (arrow).

The histology of a ***glomus jugulare tumor*** (Fig. 2.**92**) is similar to the carotid body tumor, with which it may coexist. If the glomus tumor occupies the middle ear, it can be removed via a tympanotomy or mastoidectomy approach. When the jugular foramen is involved with loss of the cranial nerves IX, X, and X (often XII from the anterior condylar foramen is also affected), the treatment is difficult. A surgical approach to the skull base is needed via the mastoid and neck, with a neurosurgical exposure if there is an intracranial extension.

If the tumor is surgically inaccessible, radiotherapy does slow the growth of an already very slow-growing tumor, and has an important place in the management, particularly in the more elderly patient. Microembolism under radiographic control of the vessels supplying the tumor is a further modality used in the treatment of these very vascular lesions, prior to surgery.

Trauma

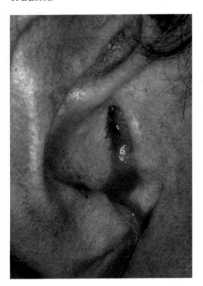

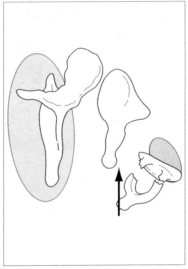

Fig. 2.**93 Bleeding.** Bleeding from the ear or a red or "blue" drum (see Fig. 2.**82**), if the tympanic membrane does not rupture, may also follow a base-of-skull fracture with bleeding into the middle ear.

Fig. 2.**94 Injury to the ear ossicles.** This may follow head injury. Dislocation of the incudostapedial joint is commonest (approx. 75%) (arrow), but fracture of the stapes crura and disruption of the stapes footplate also occur.

Barotrauma causing marked middle-ear pressure change, e. g., from diving or flying, may also disrupt the stapes footplate ligament or rupture the round window, causing perilymph fluid from the inner ear to pass into the middle ear (arrow)—a ***perilymph fistula.*** A fluctuating sensorineural hearing loss and vertigo ensue.

Fistulae often heal spontaneously, but a persistent perilymph leak needs to be sealed surgically.

Otosclerosis: Hearing Loss Due to Fixation of the Stapes Bone

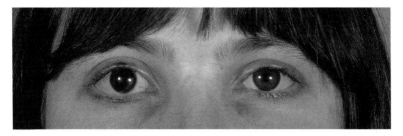

Fig. 2.**95 Otosclerosis.** This is a common cause of bilateral symmetrical conductive hearing loss in adults.

The stapes footplate is ankylosed in the oval window by thick vascular bone. This curious bony lesion is usually an isolated middle-ear focus. It may be associated, however, with **osteogenesis imperfecta tarda,** and blue sclerae are occasionally seen with *otosclerosis*, a common cause of bilateral symmetrical conductive hearing loss in adults.

Otosclerosis is familial and more common in women (otosclerotic hearing loss increases during pregnancy, which may account for the apparently higher incidence in women). Patients frequently notice paracusis, in which there is improved hearing with background noise. The cause of otosclerosis remains unknown.

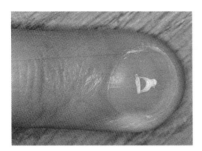

Fig. 2.**96 The stapes.** The smallest bone in the body. It is, like the other ossicles, adult size at birth.

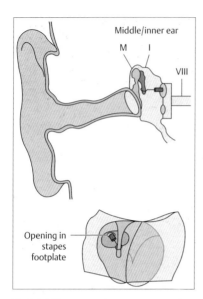

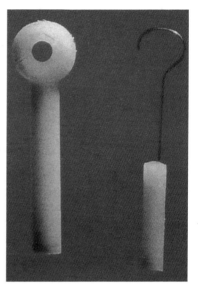

Fig. 2.**97 The stapedectomy operation.** The operation for hearing loss due to otosclerosis involves removal or perforation of the ankylosed stapes bone and replacement with a mobile prosthesis. This very successful operation was devised by John Shea of Memphis, Tennessee, United States, in 1957, and was a great advance in surgery, with good hearing achieved in over 90 % of cases.

The diagram shows the attachment of the stapes prosthesis to the long process of the incus; the distal end of the prosthesis is placed through the opening made in the ankylosed stapes footplate. The lower diagram shows the exposure of the middle ear for stapedectomy. The drum is reflected anteriorly, hinging on the long process of the malleus. The stapes superstructure and part of the footplate are removed, and the prosthesis inserted. (M: malleus; I: incus; VIII: vestibulo cochlear nerve.)

Fig. 2.**98 There are several types of prosthesis,** of which Teflon (left) and Teflon-wire are commonly used.

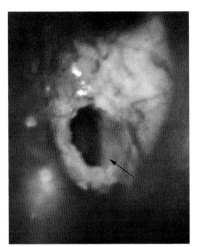

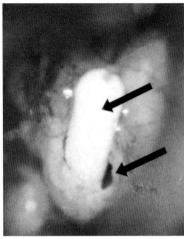

Fig. 2.**99** **Stapedectomy.** An opening is made in the fixed footplate (arrow). The laser is often used to make this opening with minimal trauma to the inner ear. The white marks to the right of this opening into the inner ear are the otoliths.

The prosthesis is attached to the long process of the incus, and the distal end of the prosthesis is placed into the inner ear.

Fig. 2.**100 A Teflon-wire prosthesis** (top arrow). The distal end is entering the inner ear through the hole in the footplate (lower arrow).

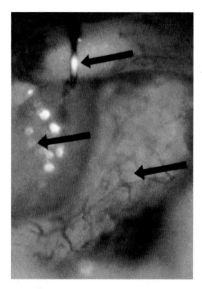

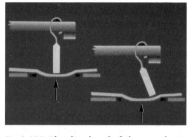

Fig. 2.**102 The distal end of the prosthesis must not only lie precisely in the stapedectomy (or stapedotomy) opening** but a "seal" is required to avoid a perilymph fistula and leakage from the inner ear fluid into the middle ear. **A vein graft** (arrows) is one of the options for this seal.

Fig. 2.**101 Fat-wire prosthesis.** The wire loop is closed on the incus (top arrow) and a fat graft (middle arrow) seals the oval window. The bone covering the facial nerve (bottom arrow). It is important for the stapedectomy prosthesis to be closed like a ring on the finger on the long process of the incus.

This ensures that the prosthesis will not slip, but also that pressure does not predispose to incus necrosis. The lentiform nodule on the incus is preserved and is a further factor ensuring that the prosthesis/incus attachment is secure.

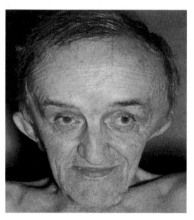

Fig. 2.**103 Conductive hearing loss very similar to otosclerosis is seen with Paget's disease.** The bony changes seen with Paget's disease, however, tend to affect the entire ossicular chain and not specifically the stapes.

Surgery for conductive hearing loss with Paget's disease is usually not advisable and hearing aids are to be preferred.

Microsurgery

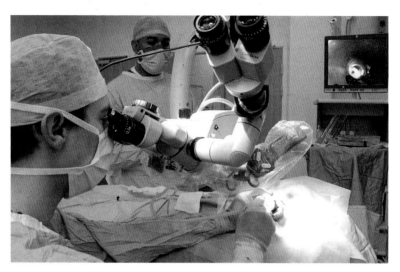

Fig. 2.**104 The middle-ear operating microscope.** Middle-ear surgery is possible because of the development of the middle-ear operating microscope. This apparatus makes the drum, ossicles, and other middle-ear structures easy to manipulate with fine instruments. The microscope is sterilized with a drape, and a camera and video camera and tutor arm can be attached.

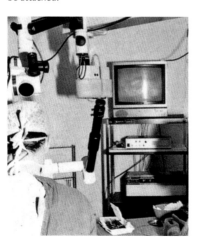

Fig. 2.**105 Operating microscope.** A TV camera can also be attached to the microscope with a monitor, giving the surgeon and observers a good operative view.

Facial Palsy

Facial palsy may follow skull fracture or facial nerve laceration near the stylomastoid foramen, and is also an uncommon complication of middle-ear surgery and superficial parotidectomy. An extensive cholesteatoma or middle-ear carcinoma may also damage the facial nerve. In the absence of a careful examination of the tympanic membrane, such a case may be wrongly diagnosed and treated as Bell's palsy. ***All facial palsies should have an otological assessment.***

Bilateral facial palsy is an interesting rarity. It is the facial asymmetry of facial palsy that is conspicuous and makes the diagnosis obvious; a bilateral facial palsy may not be so readily diagnosed.

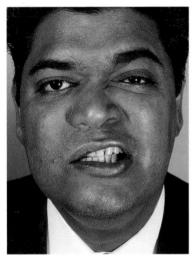

Fig. 2.**106 Bell's palsy** *is the commonest cause of facial palsy* and is a lower motor neuron lesion of the facial nerve, of unknown etiology, involving a loss of movement of facial muscles, usually total, of one side of the face. This includes the muscles of the forehead (with facial paralysis due to an upper motor neuron lesion, such as a stroke, these muscles continue to function due to cross innervation distal to the cortex).

Pain in or around the ear frequently precedes Bell's palsy, and a history of draught on the side of the face may be significant. Bell's palsy may be recurrent and associated with parotid swelling (Melkersson-Rosenthal's syndrome).

The etiology and management of Bell's palsy is controversial, although the cause is almost certainly viral.

Edema of the facial nerve near the stylomastoid foramen has been demonstrated. Most Bell's palsies recover completely and spontaneously within 6 weeks. If seen in the early stages, however, antiviral treatment and prednisolone orally should be given. Providing there is no general medical contraindication to steroids, "a" suggested dose of prednisolone is: *20 mg q. d. s. five days: 20 mg t. d. s. one day: 20 mg b.d. one day: 20 mg o. d. one day: 10 mg o. d. one day. Physiotherapy maintains tone in the muscles during recovery and also has a place in the management of Bell's palsy. Bilateral facial palsy is very rare. These cases, however, require investigation to exclude underlying disease, e. g., Lyme disease, sarcoidosis.

Functional investigations of the facial nerve branches are sometimes helpful to diagnose the level of the lesion.

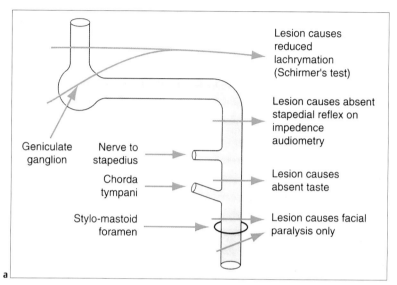

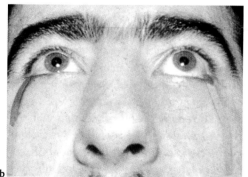

Fig. 2.**107a, b Tests of facial nerve involvement.** The level of involvement of the facial nerve in facial palsy can be determined by:

1 *Taste* (electrogustometry): if taste is absent or impaired, the lesion is proximal to the chorda tympani.

2 *Stapedial reflex* (impedance audiometry).

3 *Lacrimation* (Schirmer's test, **b**). Litmus paper is placed under the lower lid. If the facial nerve lesion is proximal to, or involves the geniculate ganglion, the tears are reduced.

These tests are reliable in traumatic section of the facial nerve to detect the level of injury. In Bell's palsy, the tests are of little value.

Electrophysiological tests provide information about prognosis. *Electroneuro-nography* is the most clinically useful test in acute complete palsy. In this test the magnitude of the action potential recorded on the affected side compared with the normal side has been shown to correlate well with a percentage of damaged axons. Although the role of intraoperative facial nerve monitoring in preventing facial nerve injury is controversial, its use has become common practice in inner ear, mastoid and parotid surgery or supervised training. Medicolegal questions may be raised should facial palsy occur when a facial nerve monitor was available but not used.

3 The Nose

Deformities

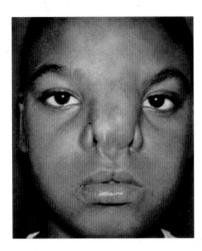

Fig. 3.1 Congenital deformities.
Abnormal fusion of the nasal processes is uncommon, and may result in varying degrees of deformity.

In this case, the nose is bifid with hypertelorism (the distance between the eyes being greatly increased). In milder cases, the bifid appearance of the nose is less marked, and may just appear as a rather "wide" nose.

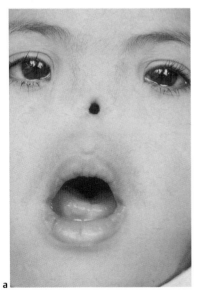

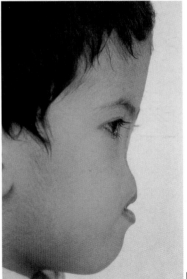

a   b

Fig. 3.**2a, b Congenital absence of the nose** is a rarity. With total atresia, this condition, as with bilateral atresia of the posterior choanae, presents an airway obstruction emergency.

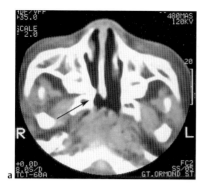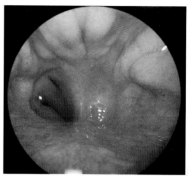

Fig. 3.3a, b Congenital atresia of one posterior choana. This congenital deformity may not present until adult life. A ***total unilateral obstruction*** from birth may cause surprisingly little trouble to the patient. If, however, the symptoms are marked, the atresia can be treated surgically with removal of the bony obstruction.

Bilateral atresia presents with dyspnea soon after birth. Immediate surgical correction is required. A membranous atresia may be perforated and dilated using metal sounds, but if the atresia is bony it must be opened with a drill, using either a transnasal or transpalatal approach. Indwelling Portex tubes are left in place for up to six weeks postoperatively to prevent a recurrence of the stenosis. ***Choanal atresia*** is well demonstrated on a computed tomograph (CT) scan, which is diagnostic. The arrow indicates the bony choanal atresia, which can be compared with the normal size. Closure of the posterior choanae with choanal atresia is well seen on this fiberoptic photograph of the postnasal space (**b**).

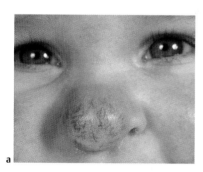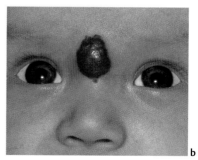

Fig. 3.4a, b Hemangiomas of the face and nose present in babies and are a cosmetic problem. Treatment is deferred, for regression in about 70 % of affected children is completed by age seven.

Parental concern or teasing of the child at school may call for earlier excision of a facial hemangioma. Surgery is also needed if regression of the lesion is incomplete. A facial hemangioma may be associated with a hemangioma elsewhere, for example in the larynx, presenting as airway obstruction and stridor.

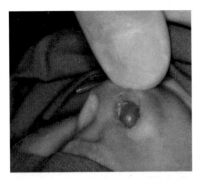

Fig. 3.**5 Nasal glioma.** This curious polypoid swelling *presents in the noses of children or babies.* A biopsy confirms the nasal glioma, which is usually an isolated entity attached to the septum. A CT scan is needed to exclude the possibility of an intracranial attachment, but this is rare. This is a benign lesion.

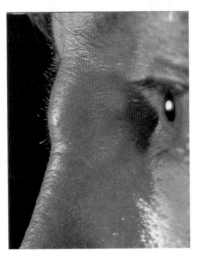

Fig. 3.**6 Dermoid.** A cystic swelling near the glabella is probably a dermoid; excision may not be straightforward. The differential diagnosis in childhood is the nasal glioma. There is commonly a sinus connecting the cyst to a punctum on the skin near the nasal tip, and there may be extension of the cyst deep to the nasal bones as far as the cribriform plate.

Cysts

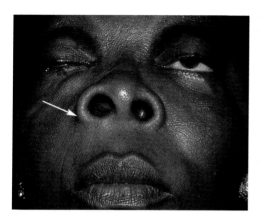

Fig. 3.7 Nasoalveolar cysts *have a constant anatomical site and spot diagnosis is possible.* Externally, there is flattening of the nasolabial fold and flaring of the alae nasi. In the anterior nares the cyst extends into the floor of the nose and displaces the inferior turbinate upwards. Excision via a sublabial incision and enucleation is the treatment. Surgical rupture of the cyst usually means incomplete removal, and predisposes to recurrence. The arrow indicates "flaring" of ala.

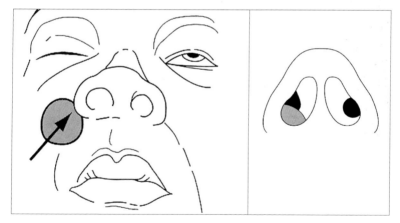

Fig. 3.8 **Nasoalveolar cysts.**

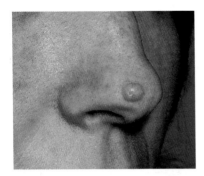

Fig. 3.9 Nasal papilloma. Benign lesions on the nose such as a mole or papilloma are common. If large, however, the obvious site on the nose necessitates excision and biopsy.

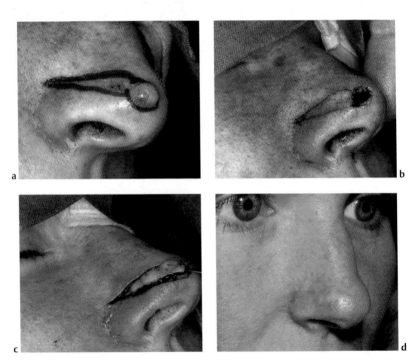

Fig. 3.10 Nasal papilloma excision. Excision is not straightforward. An elliptical excision with closure will produce an obvious nasal asymmetry, and more elaborate techniques are required to ensure a satisfactory result, e.g., an island sliding flap (**a–c**).

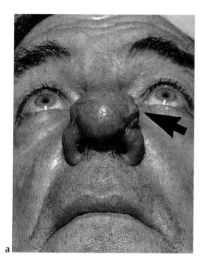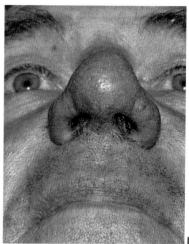

a   b

Fig. 3.**11a, b Rhinophyma**, in which the skin becomes thickened and vascular, may produce gross nasal deformity in which the skin epithelium becomes thickened and vascular. "Shaving" of the excess skin (without skin grafting) is the surgical treatment. Irregular areas of epithelium (arrow) should be sent for histology since ***basal or squamous cell carcinoma*** may occur within a rhinophyma.

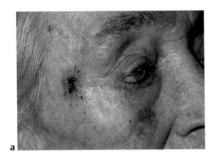

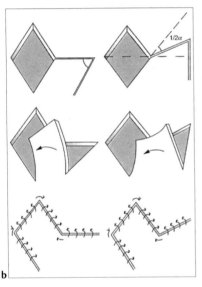

Fig. 3.**12a, b Basal cell carcinoma** (rodent cell carcinoma) are common on the nose, face, and ear. Any persistent ulcer, which may bleed, or area of induration should arouse suspicion.

Excision, radiotherapy, or laser treatment is curative for early lesions. More superficial lesions respond to fluorouracil cream. Deeply erosive basal cell carcinomas may be difficult to resect or cure. Many basal cell carcinomas require wide excision.

A simple elliptical excision leads to unnecessary scarring, which is to be avoided on the face. Incisions are made in the relaxed skin tension lines of the face and a number of flaps devised, e.g., the rhomboid as demonstrated here to minimize scarring.

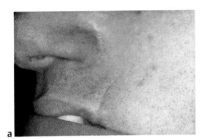

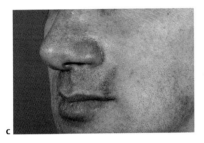

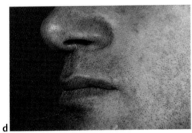

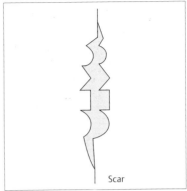

Scar

Fig. 3.**13a–d Scar revision. a** When a scar on the face is prominent, simple excision and resuturing does not always give an improved result. **b** The "breaking-up" of the line when the scar is excised makes a scar considerably less evident. Facial scars may be improved markedly with techniques such as these but complete eradication is rarely possible. **c** One month after scar revision. **d** Nine months after scar revision.

Adenoids

Persistent snoring in a child is the main symptom of enlarged adenoids. In day-time there is mouth breathing. Purulent rhinorrhea (if there is secondary sinusitis) and epistaxis also occur, with or without nasal symptoms. There is hearing loss due to otitis media with effusion, or earache from recurrent acute otitis media.

Adenoids normally regress before puberty and adults with large adenoids are rare. If an adult has nasal obstruction due to postnasal lymphoid tissue, the histology is essential to exclude a lymphoma.

Nasal obstruction may occur from birth due to large adenoids, and the baby has difficulty with bottle and breast feeding. It is occasionally necessary to remove these "congenital adenoids" in toddlers.

A conservative attitude should be taken, however, with removal of adenoids awaiting regression of the lymphoid tissue. Adenoidectomy alone is not common surgery. Tonsillar enlargement is usually also present, and is an additional cause of the upper respiratory tract obstruction and snoring.

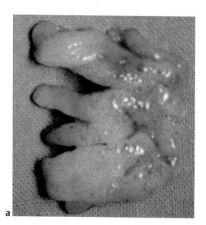
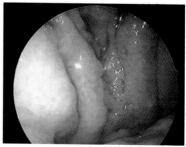

a   b

Fig. 3.**14a, b Adenoids. a** A mass of lymphoid tissue shaped like a bunch of bananas occupies the vault of the postnasal space in children. If the adenoids are large, nasal obstruction occurs. **b** Comparison of the view of the adenoids seen through the nose with an endoscope rather than with the mirror or retrograde endoscopy (see Fig. 1.**55**).

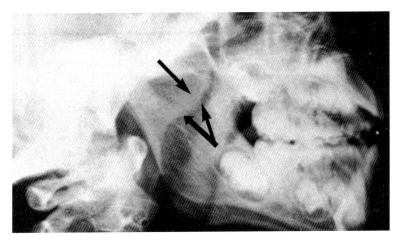

Fig. 3.15 Lateral radiograph of adenoids. The postnasal space is often difficult or impossible to see in a child, and a lateral radiograph clearly shows the size of the adenoids and degree of obstruction. In this radiograph, a small airway is present (lower arrows) despite a large adenoid shadow (upper arrow).

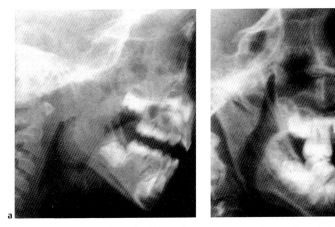

Fig. 3.16a, b Accurate lateral radiographs are necessary. A wrongly angled radiograph (**a**) is not infrequently erroneously reported as showing "large adenoids." It is not easy to maintain a child in the correct position; patience and skill are required by the radiographer. When checking the lateral radiograph for adenoids, therefore, it is essential to be sure that the lateral picture is true (**b**) before assessing the bulk of the adenoid lymphoid tissue.

Trauma

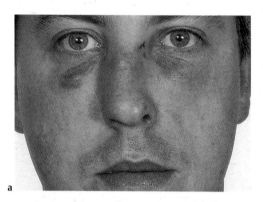

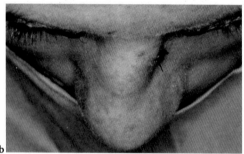

Fig. 3.**17a, b Fractured nose.** This common injury only requires treatment if the septum is dislocated or involved in hematoma, or if there is an external deviation of the nose which is of cosmetic concern to the patient (**a**: seen frontally; **b**: most obvious when examined from above). It is important to reduce nasal fractures within two weeks, lest the bones cannot be manipulated and a subsequent rhinoplasty or refracture may be necessary. Reduction, therefore, is either carried out soon after the fracture or delayed until the edema, which makes assessment of the deformity difficult, has settled (usually within four to 10 days). *Many fractured noses, however, are "chip" or undisplaced crack fractures with hematoma, and require no treatment.*

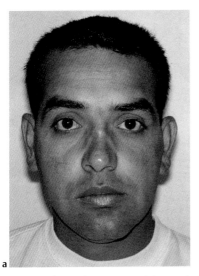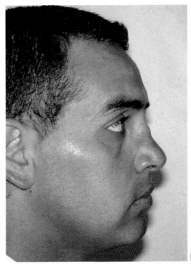

a b

Fig. 3.**18a, b Nasal injury.** Direct injury to the junction of the nasal bone and septal cartilage may cause a step deformity due to avulsion of the attachment of the upper lateral cartilages to the nasal bone. Correction requires a rhinoplasty and onlay cartilage grafting.

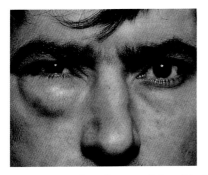

Fig. 3.**19 Surgical emphysema of the orbit.** *An alarming and unusual complication of a nasal fracture is surgical emphysema of the orbit when the patient blows the nose or sneezes.* This is due to a fracture through the ethmoidal cells and lamina papyracea, linking the nasal cavity to the orbit. There is no cause for alarm, and if care is taken not to inflate the orbit, spontaneous healing follows. ***The characteristic crepitus on palpation is diagnostic.*** A facial injury that has caused a nasal fracture may also have involved the maxilla and anterior cranial fossa (with cerebrospinal fluid rhinorrhea), and ***precautions should be taken to exclude such an associated fracture as well as any possible injury to the eye.***

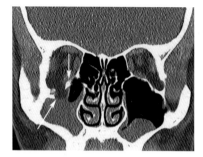

Fig. 3.**20 A "blow-out" fracture** with fat herniation into the maxillary antrum occurs with the sudden rise in intraorbital pressure after blunt trauma to the orbit and nose. The upper arrow shows the bony defect through which the fat (lower arrow) prolapses.

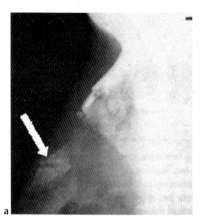

a

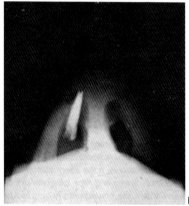

b

Fig. 3.**21a, b Radiographs of nasal bones showing complete separation of one bone.** In this case, the nasal bone radiograph shows some obvious and significant injury. In most instances, however, the radiographs for a fractured nose are of little practical value, although they may be of medicolegal significance.

Complications of a Fractured Nose

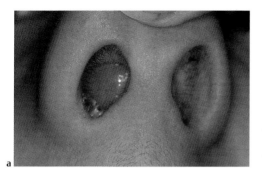

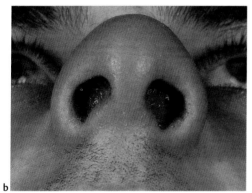

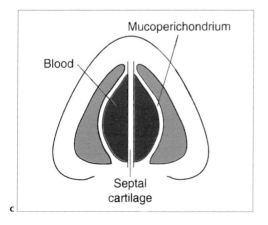

Fig. 3.**22a–c A septal hematoma following trauma to the nose.** Blood collects under the subperichondrium on both sides, causing "ballooning" of the septum and total nasal obstruction. *If the nasal obstruction is total, early drainage of the hematoma is required.* A warning must be given preoperatively that nasal saddling of the dorsum may ensue, the hematoma having led to necrosis of the septal cartilage. *Septal swelling with partial nasal obstruction usually settles spontaneously, and drainage is not necessary.* The hematoma, if left, may become infected. Pain and malaise accompany the total nasal blockage. Draining is necessary, and saddling is then common (see Fig. 3.**24**).

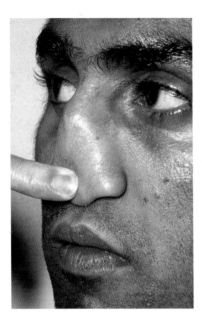

Fig. 3.**23 A septal hematoma** may lead to lack of septal support to the nasal dorsum. With infected hematomas loss of support is common.

Rhinoplasty

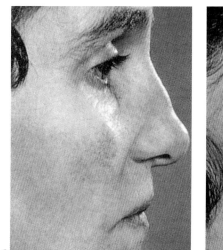
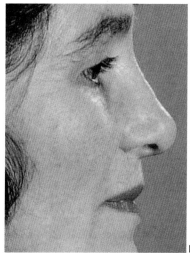

Fig. 3.**24a, b Nasal saddling.** Minimal saddling, as in this patient (**a**) may accentuate a previous nasal hump. Simple lowering of the nasal bones restores the appearance of a normal nose (**b**).

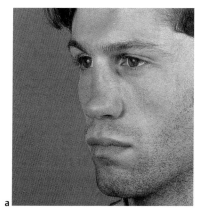
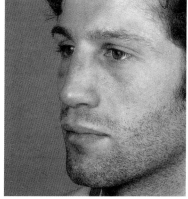

Fig. 3.**25a, b A saddle nasal deformity following trauma, and a septal hematoma.** This was repaired with cartilage graft taken from the concha of the ear.

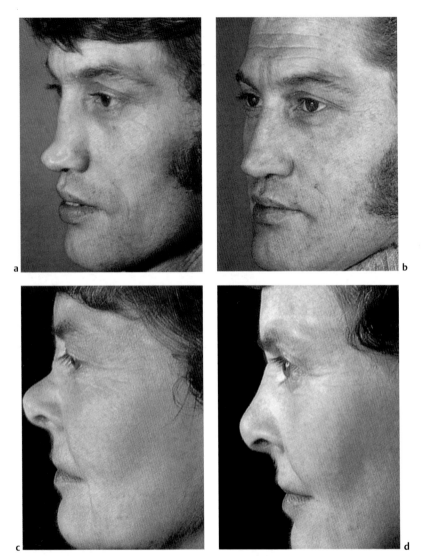

Fig. 3.**26a–d Grafts.** With more severe saddling, a graft is needed to restore the nasal contour. Cartilage, bone, or a synthetic are alternative grafting materials.

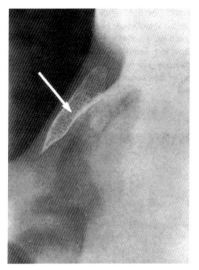

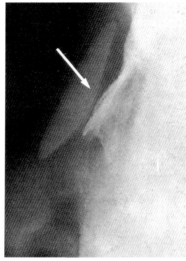

Fig. 3.**27 Iliac crest bone graft.** An iliac crest bone graft (arrow) used for a saddle deformity is demonstrable on this radiograph.

Fig. 3.**28 Synthetic graft.** A synthetic graft (silastic) seen on radiograph (arrow), is also used to correct nasal saddling.

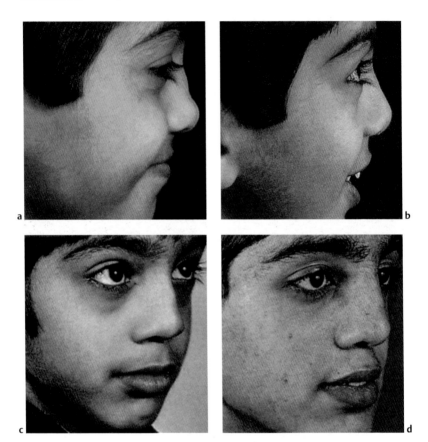

Fig. 3.**29a–d Septal hematomas in childhood.** Septal hematomas are not uncommon in children, and may follow trauma or be spontaneous, in which case a blood dyscrasia needs to be excluded. The parents should be warned that the development of the nose may be retarded, and *may lead to a "small" nose in adult life.* In the past, surgical correction was left until the nose was fully grown at age 16–17, but it is now apparent that grafting of these saddle deformities in childhood will lead to more normal nasal development. **a** A childhood saddle deformity before grafting (age seven). **b** After grafting (age seven). **c** Age 11. **d** A normal nose and not an infantile nose has developed as a result of grafting in childhood (age 19).

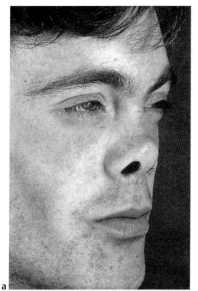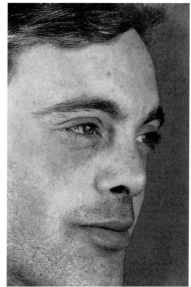

a   b

Fig. 3.**30a, b Nasal plastic surgery. a** A small infantile nose following a septal abscess in childhood. **b** Nasal plastic surgery using cartilage and composite ear grafts gives significant improvement.

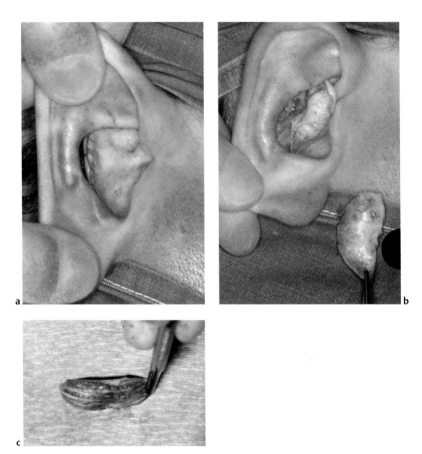

Fig. 3.**31a–e Cartilage grafts** are taken from the concha of the ear (**a–c**), leaving no aural deformity. The cartilage grafts are placed in the nose as shown (**d, e**).

Fig. 3.**31d, e** ▶

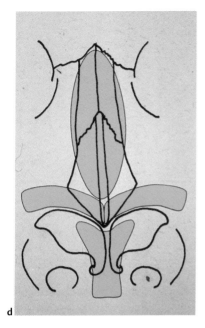

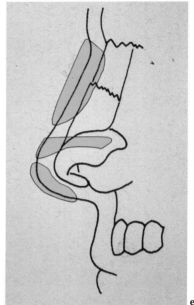

d

e

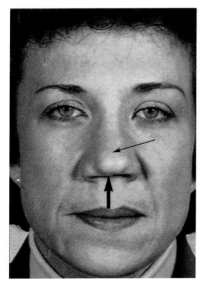

Fig. 3.**32 Retraction of the columella.** Retraction of the columella (lower arrow), loss of tip support, and saddling (arrow) of the nose are also complications of a septal hematoma, and common if infection occurs.

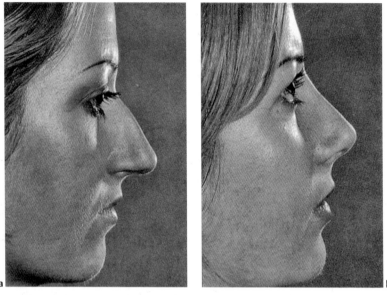

a

b

Fig. 3.**33a–f Rhinoplasty.** The appearance of a nose with a congenital or traumatic hump of the nasal bones can be improved with rhinoplasty (**a–d**). A deviated nose may be straightened (**e, f**).

Fig. 3.**33c–f** ▶

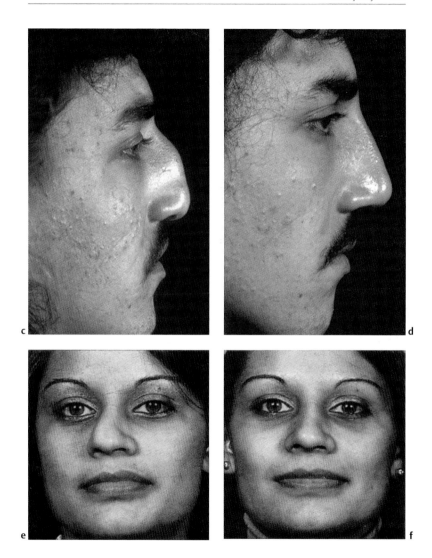

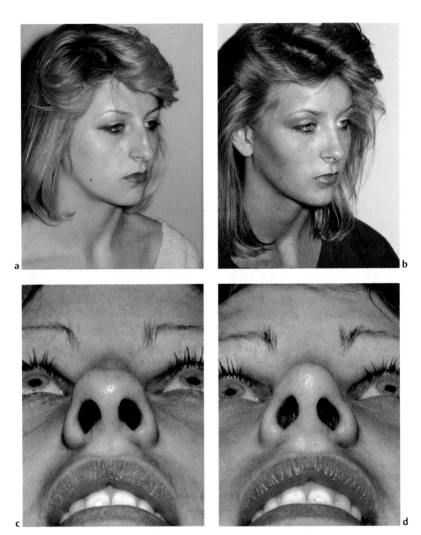

Fig. 3.**34a–f Nasal tip rhinoplasty.** Bulbous or bifid nasal tips can be modified (**c, d**). Incisions for rhinoplasty are within the nasal vestibule and access to the nasal bones, cartilages, and septum may be obtained with an intranasal (or external, see Fig. 3.**44**) approach.

Fig. 3.**34e, f** ▶

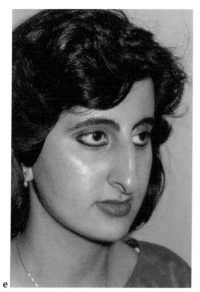

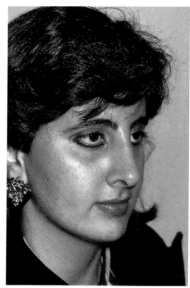

e

f

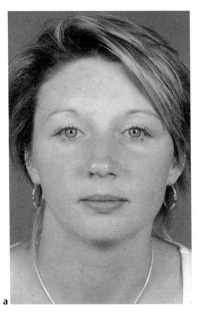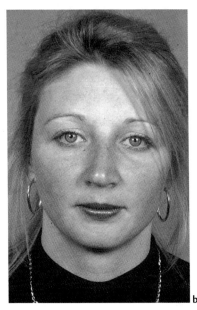

a
b

Fig. 3.**35a, b** **Bifidity of nasal tip** is corrected with narrowing and reduction of the alar cartilage.

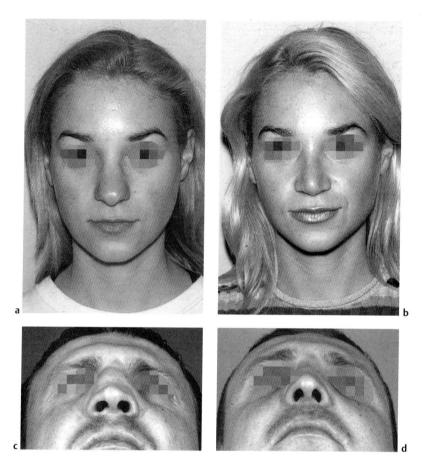

Fig. 3.**36a–d The wide nose** may be congenital (**a, b**) or caused by trauma (**c, d**)—usually repeated trauma. Rhinoplasty involves excision of excess nasal bone and infracture of the bone.

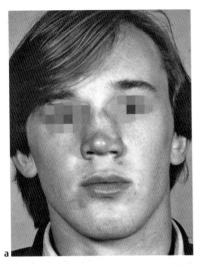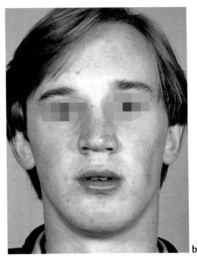

a   b

Fig. 3.**37a, b** **The deviated nose** is usually caused by trauma. If there is a septal injury, saddling and deviation may result. Conchal cartilage grafts and refracture of the nasal bones
are necessary.

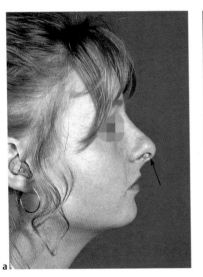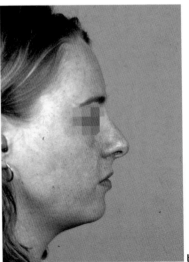

a   b

Fig. 3.**38a, b** **The low columella** (arrow) is often due to excess nasal septal cartilage, and excision of this cartilage is effective surgery.

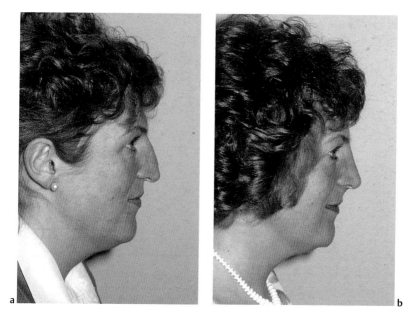

Fig. 3.**39a, b The retracted columella** is often associated with past septal trauma. A large cartilage graft, e.g., conchal, is needed for correction.

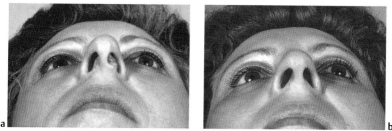

Fig. 3.**40a, b The wide columella** is not easy to correct. It may be caused by large feet of the medial crura of the nasal cartilages. Rhinoplasty involves excision or suturing of these cartilages.

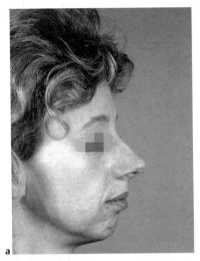
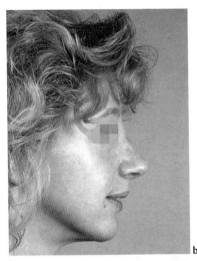

a   b

Fig. 3.**41a, b The prominent nose** may be accentuated by a receding chin. The esthetic improvement of the rhinoplasty is improved if mentoplasty is also carried out.

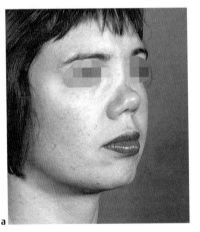
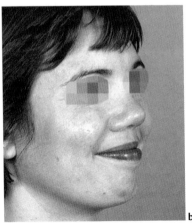

a   b

Fig. 3.**42a Wegener's granuloma** (p. 150) may cause septal necrosis and nasal saddling. **b** Rhinoplasty with graft to nasal dorsum.

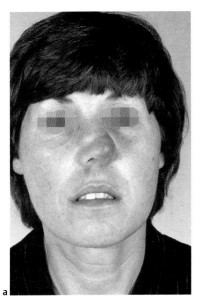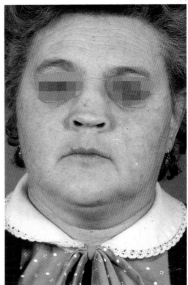

a b

Fig. 3.**43a, b** **The possibility of pathology other than congenital or traumatic must be remembered when diagnosing nasal deformity.** *Sarcoid* not uncommonly presents with nasal deformity (**a**) and *relapsing polychondritis* may also involve nasal septal cartilage and present with widening and saddling (**b**).

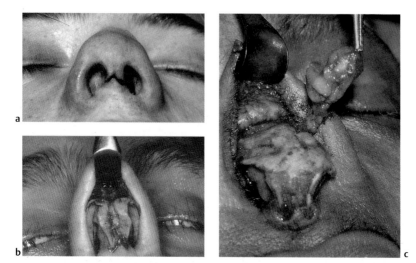

Fig. 3.**44a–c External rhinoplasty.** A transverse incision across the columella (**a**, with a "notch" to give a minimally perceptible scar) enables the skin of the nose to be elevated superiorly with exposure of all the underlying structures (**b**).

This rhinoplasty approach is used for many nasal deformities. It also enables lesions on the dorsum of the nose to be excised without an obvious overlying scar. The lesion being removed here is a nasal sinus (**c**).

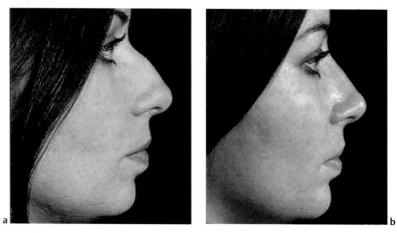

Fig. 3.**45a, b Mentoplasty.** The improvement with rhinoplasty in this case has been accentuated by mentoplasty (see Fig. 3.**46**).

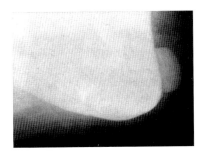

Fig. 3.**46 A silastic implant** has been inserted adjacent to the mandible. A receding chin is not to be overlooked in a patient seeking rhinoplasty, for it accentuates the nasal deformity, and mentoplasty gives a subtle but striking improvement in appearance.

This implant may be introduced either by an external submental incision or on intraoral incision via the mucosa of the buccal sulcus.

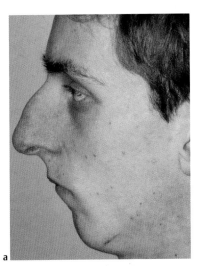

a

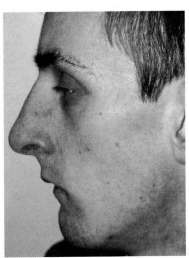

b

Fig. 3.**47a–c Marked mandibular underdevelopment** (**a**) in which a mandibular advancement to restore dental occlusion as well as the esthetics was combined with a rhinoplasty (**b**). The radiograph (**c**) shows the sliding advancement and wiring of the mandibular bone.

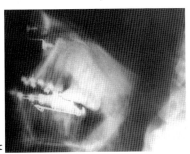

c

Deviated Nasal Septum

A congenital or traumatic dislocation of the septal cartilage into one nasal fossa causes unilateral nasal obstruction. If the obstruction is marked, or complicated by recurrent sinusitis, a septal correction is effective surgery.

The time-honored operation for this is **a submucous resection (SMR)**, but a **septoplasty** in which cartilage is preserved and repositioned—rather than removed—is now used. The SMR operation involves removal of much of the septal cartilage and loss of nasal support with saddling, and septal perforations are occasional complications.

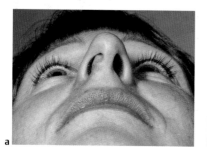
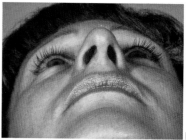

a   b

Fig. 3.**48a, b Deviated nasal septum into the columella.** With caudal dislocation of the septum, an obvious deformity is coupled with nasal obstruction (**a**). Repositioning or excision of the septal dislocation is necessary to improve the appearance and airway (**b**).

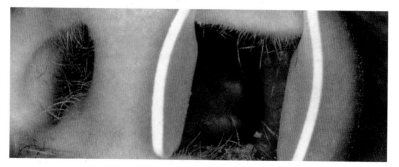

Fig. 3.**49 Deviated nasal septum.** Deviated nasal septum with a spur of septal cartilage and maxillary bone occluding the inferior meatus and causing nasal obstruction.

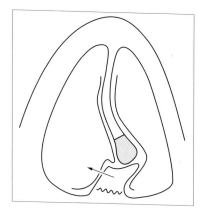

Fig. 3.50 Septoplasty technique.

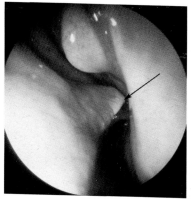

Fig. 3.**51 A posterior spur (arrow) on a deviated nasal septum seen with the endoscope.** Most septal deviations can be seen with a speculum but are seen with greater clarity with the endoscope, and the application of a nasal vasoconstrictor to the mucosa.

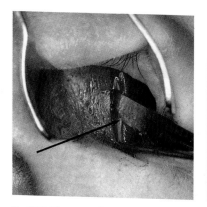

Fig. 3.**52 The septoplasty operation.** An incision through the nasal mucosa and cartilage with elevation of the mucoperichondrium (arrow) gives access to the septal cartilage, which is partially resected and repositioned.

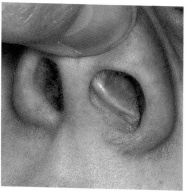

Fig. 3.**53 Deviated nasal septum in a child.** The diagnosis is obvious without the use of a nasal speculum. Elevation of the infantile nasal tip suffices to give a clear view of the anterior nares.

Perforations of the Nasal Septum

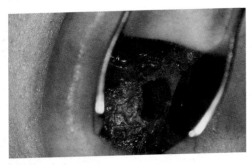

Fig. 3.**54** A perforation of the nasal septum. This may not give rise to any symptoms, and be a chance finding on examination. Crusting usually occurs, however, causing nasal obstruction and discomfort, with episodes of scanty epistaxis.

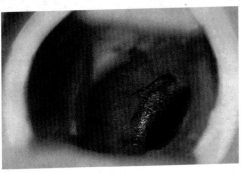

Fig. 3.**55 Prominent blood vessels** appearing on the margin of the perforation, leading to epistaxis. *A whistling noise on breathing is another symptom.*

The symptoms of crusting, bleeding, and a whistling noise on breathing may call for surgical closure. An external approach is often needed for access to elevate mucosal flaps from the perforation margin to be rotated over a cartilage or fascial graft. The success rate with small or moderate sized perforations is about 70%, but with large perforations over 2–3 cm surgical closure is often not successful.

Perforations may result from repeated trauma to the septum (e.g., nose picking). An inadvertent tear of the nasal mucous membrane on both sides during septal surgery is another cause of perforation. Cocaine snorters risk a nasal vestibulitis (pp. 146–147) and a septal perforation. Skin necrosis with loss of the nasal columella may also occur. Those working with chrome are susceptible to septal perichondritis and a perforation.

Destruction of the vomer and ethmoid bone accounts for a posterior septal perforation, and may be due to a gumma (syphilis).

It is fortunate that many perforations are symptom-free, because surgical repair, particularly of large perforations, is not easy. An external rhinoplasty approach may be needed to raise mucosal flaps adjacent to the perforation, which are rotated and sutured over a cartilage or fascial graft. Plastic flanged prostheses have been tried to seal the perforation but may extrude or be uncomfortable.

Inflammation

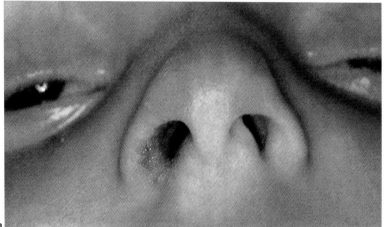

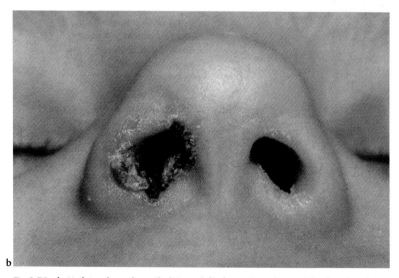

Fig. 3.**56a, b Unilateral nasal vestibulitis and discharge** (purulent and fetid in **a**) is almost always *diagnostic of a foreign body in a child's nose*, as is *unilateral nasal vestibulitis* alone (**b**).

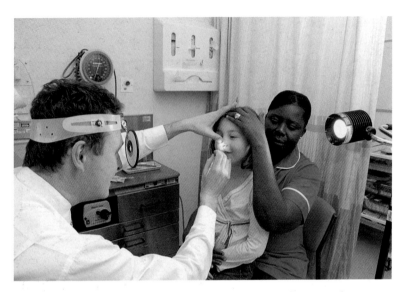

Fig. 3.57 Removal of a foreign body. Removal frequently can be managed as an out-patient, when it is necessary to hold the child securely while a probe or hook is placed posterior to the foreign body. Forceps frequently push the foreign body posteriorly, and thus should be avoided. A general anesthetic is necessary if the foreign body is impacted or inaccessible.

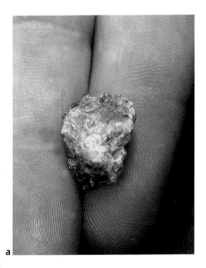

a

Fig. 3.58a, b Rhinolith. A foreign body that is ignored accumulates a calcareous deposit and presents years later as a fetid, stony, hard mass—a rhinolith (**a**). This is well demonstrated radiologically (**b**), and a rhinolith may become large, eroding the lateral wall and floor of the nose.

Although at first sight appearing easy to remove, the impaction may be extremely firm, particularly with the larger rhinoliths.

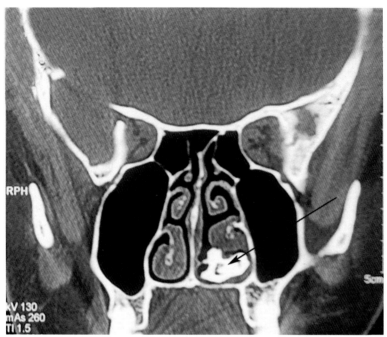

b

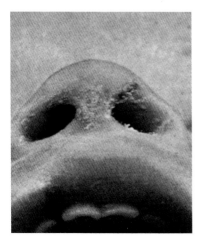

Fig. 3.**59 Vestibulitis.** When nasal discharge and skin infection affect both nostrils, a vestibulitis (an eczema of the vestibular skin) is the diagnosis. Cleaning and causing trauma with the finger nail, removal of nasal vibrissae, and cocaine snorting predispose to this condition.

Advice and use of an antibiotic ointment, e.g., Bactroban, is usually curative. The nasal swab usually grows a staphylococcus.

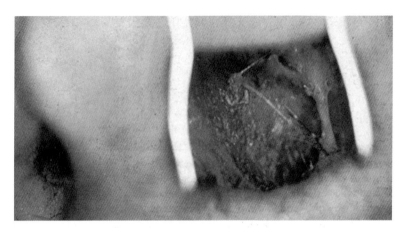

Fig. 3.**60 Vestibulitis** *presents as crusting and irritation in the anterior nares with resulting nasal obstruction.* Examination shows excoriated vestibular skin and septal mucous membrane. *Rubbing or over-diligent cleaning of the nose by the patient usually causes vestibulitis,* particularly if, as in this case, the septum is deviated anteriorly and impinges on the lateral wall of the nose. Advice and the use of antibiotic and corticosteroid ointment are effective in controlling vestibulitis. Correction of the septum may be necessary.

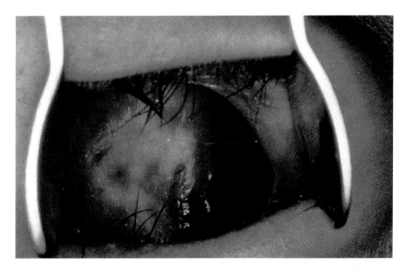

Fig. 3.**61 Nasal vestibulitis with squamous epithelium replacing the mucosa.** A deviation of the septum has predisposed to a chronic vestibulitis. Digital irritation, or the ***use of cocaine***, which may also lead to a septal perforation, may underlie this problem.

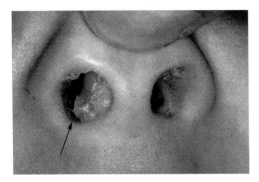

Fig. 3.**62 Vestibulitis in a child overlying a grossly deviated anterior septum** (arrow). Septal surgery is avoided in children, but cases in which the obstruction is gross require a conservative septoplasty. Excessive cartilage resection may retard nasal growth, predisposing to saddling or an infantile nose (Fig 3.**30a**).

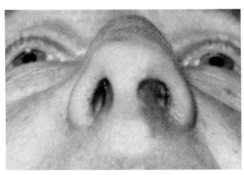

Fig. 3.**63 Vestibulitis.** Painful crusting of the nasal vestibule and anterior nares may be a simple eczematous type of skin lesion which settles with a topical antibiotic and steroid ointment. There should, however, be an awareness that this vestibulitis may be a *granuloma,* or part of the manifestation of systemic disease such as polyarteritis nodosa or systemic lupus erythematosus. A further possibility is an "irritative" vestibulitis from *cocaine snuff,* or *columellar carcinoma,* as in this case.

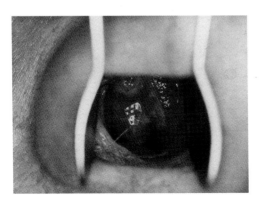

Fig. 3.**64 Granular rhinitis.** Granulation tissues in the nose requires biopsy. *Sarcoidosis* not infrequently involves the upper respiratory tract mucosa of the nasal fossae and larynx. In the nose the granulations are pale, but tuberculosis, malignant granuloma, and neoplasia are among the differential diagnoses.

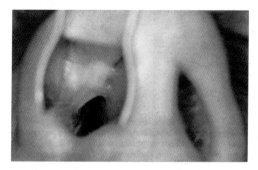

Fig. 3.**65 Nasal adhesion.** Adhesion or synechiae may follow nasal trauma (including surgical trauma) and bridge the lateral wall of the nose, frequently from the inferior turbinate to the septum, causing nasal obstruction. Recurrence follows surgical division of the larger adhesions unless an indwelling silastic splint is left in situ until mucosa underlying the adhesion regenerates.

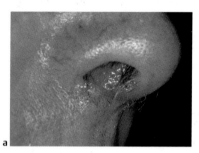

a

Fig. 3.**66a, b   Furuncles and cellulitis of the columella (a).** These may spread to involve the skin of the nose and face (**b**). Treatment is with systemic penicillin.

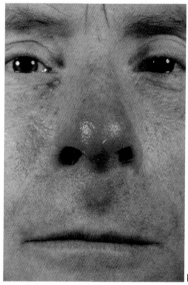

b

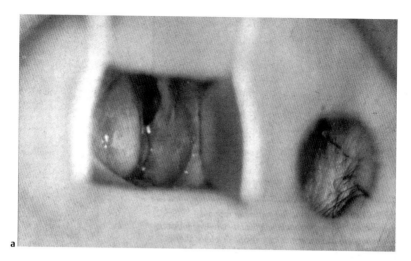

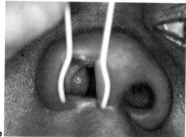

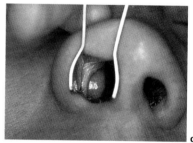

Fig. 3.**67a–c Acute rhinitis.** In the ***common cold***, the nasal mucous membrane is edematous, so the inferior turbinate abuts against the septum to result in obstruction and an excess of mucous which causes the running nose.

A similar appearance is seen in ***nasal allergy***, either "seasonal hay fever" or perennial allergy, but the edematous turbinate mucous membrane appears ***gray*** (**c**) rather than red (**b**). A persistent purulent nasal discharge usually means that there is a sinusitis. Corticosteroid nasal sprays for nasal allergy reduce the obstruction, rhinorrhea, and sneezing that characterize both seasonal and perennial nasal allergy. Skin tests to detect specific allergens are of use with grass pollen and house dust allergy related to the house dust mite.

Nasal sprays, along with allergen avoidance where possible, and oral antihistamines without sedative side effects are the first lines of treatment for nasal allergy. This management of nasal allergy is preferable to desensitization, as there is an increased awareness and concern regarding anaphylactic shock.

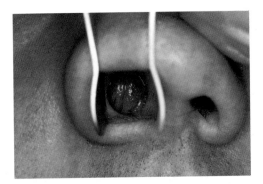

Fig. 3.**68 Chronic rhinitis.** The turbinate mucous membrane frequently reacts to irritants, whether tobacco, excessive use of vasoconstrictor drops, or atmospheric irritants, by enlarging. Thickened red inferior turbinates are seen adjacent to the septum, limiting the airway. *Nasal obstruction, either intermittent or persistent, with a postnasal discharge of mucus ("postnasal drip") are the symptoms of chronic rhinitis.* This is the condition most frequently labeled by the patient as "catarrh" or "sinus trouble."

If the changes due to chronic rhinitis are irreversible, i.e., the nasal obstruction persists when the irritants are removed, it is probable that minor surgery to reduce the turbinates in size will be necessary.

A nasal corticosteroid spray and nonsedating oral antihistamines help, but vasoconstrictor drops have no place in the treatment of chronic rhinitis and their constant use is a cause of **rhinitis medicamentosa**.

Rhinitis frequently coexists with asthma (the upper and lower respiratory tract sharing a common epithelium), and about 30% of those with rhinitis have asthma. (About 80% of asthmatics have rhinitis.)

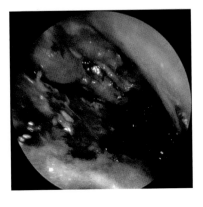

Fig. 3.**69 Wegener's granuloma.** An endoscopic view of the granulomatous tissue seen on nasal endoscopy. Wegener's granuloma is a rare autoimmune inflammatory disease which often presents with nasal symptoms of obstruction, crusting, and epistaxis. Damage to the septum may lead to a saddle deformity (Figs. 3.**24**–3.**26**).

The granulomas may be limited to the nose, but the respiratory tract may be involved along with a generalized vasculitis and glomerulonephritis. The condition is characterized by periods of remission, and treatment with oral steroids and cytotoxic drugs has dramatically improved the prognosis of a previously fatal condition.

In most inflammatory conditions of the nasal mucous membrane, there is an excess of mucus. An atrophy of the mucosa and mucous glands with fetid crusting of wide nasal fossae, however, is seen with *atrophic rhinitis*. This is uncommon and idiopathic. It may be an isolated nasal condition, part of *Wegener's granuloma*, or disseminated lupus erythematosus. There is also a phase of atrophic nasal crusting in **rhinoscleroma**.

Nasal surgery in which there is excessive resection of nasal tissue and mucosa also predisposes to atrophic crusting.

Acute Maxillary Sinusitis

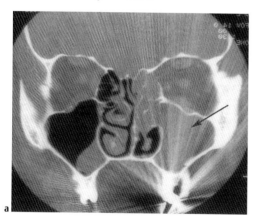

Fig. 3.**70a A CT scan showing total opacity of the left antrum and ethmoids due to infection (arrow).**

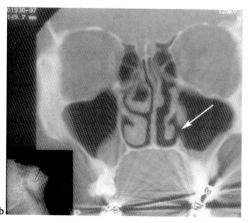

b Clearing and a return to a normal CT scan of an infected maxillary and ethmoidal sinuses following *intranasal antrostomy* (arrow). In this instance the antrostomy (or opening into the maxillary antrum), has been made through the inferior meatus. It is more commonly made through the middle meatus.

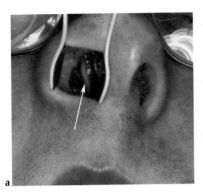
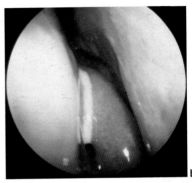

Fig. 3.**71a, b** **Maxillary sinusitis with pus** (**a**, arrow) adjacent to the middle turbinate issuing into the middle meatus, seen with the endoscope (**b**).

Acute Maxillary Sinusitis is a common complication of a head cold. If a head cold persists beyond four to five days with continued nasal obstruction, purulent rhinorrhea, and headache, the probable diagnosis is maxillary sinusitis. Apical infection of the teeth related to the antrum or an oroantral fistula following dental extraction also cause maxillary sinusitis, as may trauma with bleeding into the antrum or barotrauma.

Frontal or facial pain may be referred to the upper teeth; nasal obstruction and purulent rhinorrhea are the other symptoms. The antrum is opaque on sinus X-ray (see p.34) and on computed tomography (CT; Fig.3.**70a**). There may be tenderness over the sinus, but swelling is rare. Pus is seen issuing from the middle meatus (Fig.3.**71a**, arrow).

Acute infection may less commonly affect the ethmoid, frontal, and sphenoid sinuses. Systemic antibiotics, a vasoconstrictor spray, or drops and inhalations are usually curative for acute sinusitis. A persistent maxillary sinusitis, however, requires surgery.

Although frontal headache, and less commonly pain over the cheek, are characteristic of maxillary sinusitis, very severe pain suggests either a complication of the sinusitis, or a neuralgic cause for the pain. ***Migrainous neuralgia (cluster headaches)*** characterized by episodes of frontal pain which increase in severity reaching the level of extremely severe pain, which then regresses. Such a history, ***without nasal symptoms***, suggests a diagnosis of ***migrainous neuralgia*** and further investigation is needed.

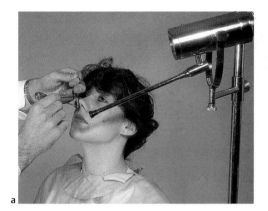

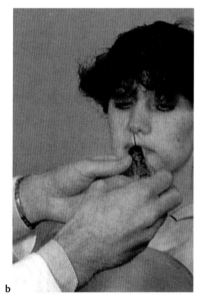

Fig. 3.**72a, b An antral washout** may be needed, albeit rarely today, for a persistent maxillary sinusitis. This involves inserting a trocar and cannula under the inferior turbinate, and puncturing the lateral wall of the nose through the maxillary process of the thin inferior turbinate bone, to enter the antrum. Water is irrigated through the cannula, and the pus emerges through the maxillary ostium.

An acutely infected maxillary sinus must not be washed out until medical treatment has controlled the acute phase. Cavernous sinus thrombosis remains a danger. The bad reputation that antral washout has for pain is not justified if a good local anesthetic and gentle technique are used.

Recurrent attacks of acute maxillary sinusitis may require operation. *A permanent intranasal opening into the antrum is made either in the middle or inferior meatus (intranasal antrostomy).* This operation is also effective for those cases of acute sinusitis that fail to respond to conservative treatment and antral washouts.

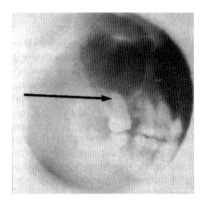

Fig. 3.**73   Dental sinusitis.** The apices of the molar teeth may be extremely close to the antral mucosal lining. The upper wisdom tooth apparent on this radiograph (arrow), if infected, would be likely to cause maxillary sinusitis or, if removed, would be clearly at risk for causing an oroantral fistula.

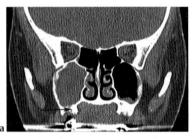

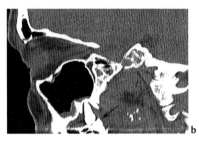

a   b

Fig. 3.**74a, b   Oroantral fistula. a** Removal of a molar tooth resulted in an oroantral fistula (arrow). **b** The root of this unerupted tooth (arrow) is seen penetrating the floor of the maxillary antrum.

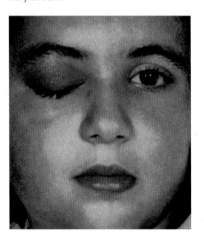

Fig. 3.**75   Orbital cellulitis.** Complications of acute sinusitis confined to the antrum are rare. A severe maxillary sinusitis, however, usually involves the ethmoid and frontal sinuses. Infection spreading via the lamina papyracea or floor of the frontal sinus leads to an orbital cellulitis. A CT scan is essential in these cases to define the extent of infection *and to exclude frontal lobe involvement*.

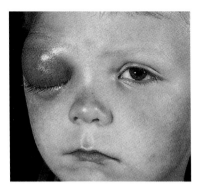

Fig. 3.**76 An orbital abscess**, requiring external drainage, may form. Meningitis or brain abscess may also follow the spread of infection from the roof of the ethmoid, frontal, or sphenoid sinus to the anterior cranial fossa.

Infection associated with a rapidly growing neoplasm, such as a ***rhabdomyosarcoma***, is the differential diagnosis in this case.

Chronic Sinusitis

Chronic sinusitis may develop from incomplete resolution of an acute infection. The onset, however, may be insidious and secondary to nasal obstruction (e. g., due to a deviated septum, nasal polyps, or, in children, to enlarged adenoids). Apical infection of the teeth related to the antra can also cause chronic sinusitis.

Purulent rhinorrhea, nasal obstruction, and headache are the main symptoms of chronic sinusitis. Pus in the middle meatus with radiographic opacity of the sinus are confirmatory of infection. Pus confined to the antrum rarely gives complications, but often there is a spread of infection to the ethmoids and frontal sinuses. It is not common for frontal and ethmoid sinusitis to occur without maxillary sinusitis. Pus in the frontal and ethmoid sinus, as with acute infections, may spread to involve the orbit and brain. Obstruction of the sinus ostium may lead to encysted collection of mucus within the sinus—a ***mucocele***.

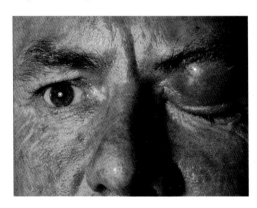

Fig. 3.**77 A mucocele**. The frontal sinus is commonly affected, and erosion of the roof of the orbit leads to orbital displacement downwards and laterally.

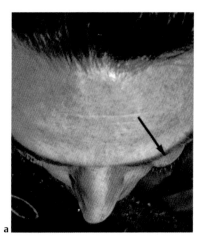
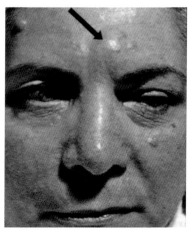

Fig. 3.**78a, b A mucocele.** Proptosis also occurs with mucoceles, and is best confirmed by examination from above (**a**, arrow). The frontal sinus wall may be eroded both posteriorly and anteriorly. An eroded anterior wall results in a fluctuant swelling on the forehead (**b**, arrow). In this case, there is also orbital displacement and proptosis.

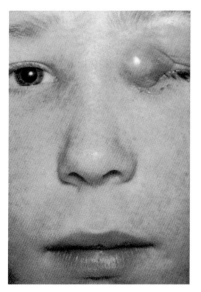

Fig. 3.**79 Lateral displacement of the orbit.** This occurs with a mucocele arising in the ethmoid sinus, and is usually accompanied by a swelling of the medial canthus. In this case, the mucocele is infected—a **pyocele**.

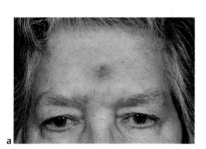
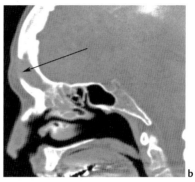

Fig. 3.**80a, b Pott's puffy tumor** is an uncommon complication of chronic frontal sinusitis where *osteomyelitis* of the frontal bone is associated with a subperiosteal abscess. "Puffy" swelling of the forehead is seen (**a**); the CT scan shows erosion of the frontal sinus (**b**, arrow) as a result of osteomyelitis.

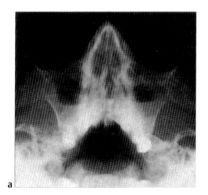
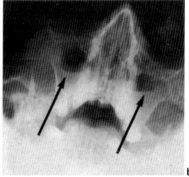

Fig. 3.**81a, b Maxillary sinus radiographs.** In acute and chronic maxillary sinusitis, a fluid level may be seen on radiography. A tilted view is taken to confirm the presence of fluid (**b**, arrows). A thickened or rather "straight" mucous membrane may look like a fluid level, as may a bony shadow if the radiograph is wrongly angled.

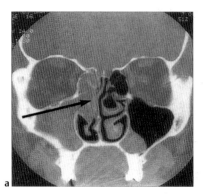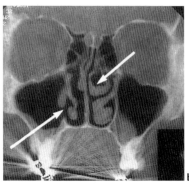

a   b

Fig. 3.**82a, b CT scans to show the sinuses.** CT scans give a much more detailed picture of the maxillary, ethmoid, frontal, and sphenoid sinuses. They are routine when endoscopic sinus surgery is anticipated, and are also of additional help to the plain sinus radiograph for diagnosis. CT scans, however, involve considerably more radiation to the orbit and are expensive. Opacity of the ethmoid sinuses characteristic of infection is seen (**a**, arrow). Also seen is an air cell in the middle turbinate (concha bullosa; **b**, upper arrow) and a right intranasal antrostomy into the maxillary sinus (**b**, lower arrow).

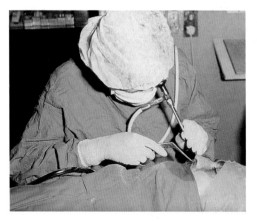

Fig. 3.**83   Endoscopic sinus surgery.** In cases of persistent sinusitis that do not respond to medical treatment, endoscopic sinus surgery is now successful in curing most cases. The improvement of instruments and techniques for nasal and sinus surgery enable biopsies of antral mucosa, excision of nasal cysts and foreign bodies in the antrum, e.g., a misplaced apical dental filling, to be dealt with via the sinus endoscope.

The Caldwell-Luc operation (Fig. 3.**85**) and radical or "open" surgery for chronic frontal sinus infections are now a rarity.

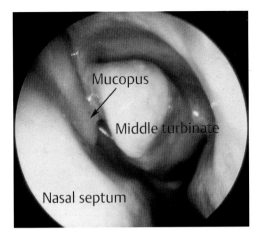

Fig. 3.**84 View through the sinus endoscope.**

Mucopus

Middle turbinate

Nasal septum

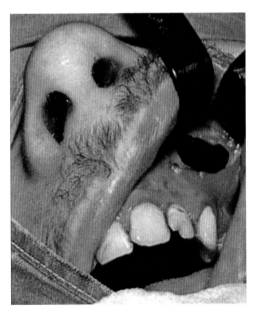

Fig. 3.**85 The Caldwell-Luc operation** in which the antrum is opened with a sublabial antrostomy, the antral mucous membrane removed, and an intranasal antrostomy is made. The Caldwell–Luc operation, previously commonly carried out, is rare. Antibiotics, endoscopic sinus surgery, and a possible change in the nature of the sinus disease account for this.

Polyps

Nasal polyps are a common cause of nasal obstruction, and may cause *anosmia*. They are benign and do *not* present with bleeding. Examination shows a gray pendulous *opalescent* swelling arising from the ethmoid. A polyp is very different in appearance from the red inferior turbinate adjacent to it.

Polyps may be solitary or multiple, often extending from the nasal vestibule to the posterior choana. They are usually bilateral. Nasal polyps may become extremely large, causing expansion of the nasal bones and alae nasi. A nasal polyp which is ulcerated and bleeds is probably malignant.

Nasal polyps result from a distension of an area of nasal mucous membrane with intercellular fluid. They are due to a hypersensitivity reaction in the mucous membrane, but may also result from sinus infection. Obstruction of the sinuses by polyps, however, may lead to a secondary sinusitis, and a sinus radiograph is a routine investigation.

Small nasal polyps may cause little in the way of symptoms and may be chance findings. Usually, however, polyps extend and enlarge, and present with nasal obstruction. They do regress with corticosteroid nose drops and sprays, but in many instances, surgical removal either under local or general anesthesia is necessary.

Nasal polyps in children or young adults, particularly if recurrent and associated with upper respiratory tract infections, suggest *cystic fibrosis*. In this condition the mucosal cilia of the respiratory tract are poorly motile (*ciliary dyskinesia*). (The young adult [Fig. 3.**90a**] with nasal bone expansion from extensive nasal polypi was found on further investigation to have cystic fibrosis.)

Nasal polyps tend to recur, and in some instances may be a recurrent lifelong problem, for example, those with the well-recognized Samter's *triad* of *recurrent nasal polypi, asthma, and aspirin hypersensitivity*.

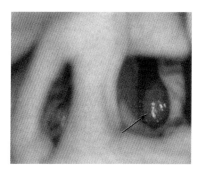

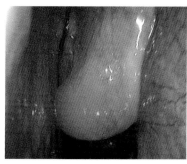

Fig. 3.**86 Nasal polyp** (arrow).

Fig. 3.**87 Nasal polyps as seen through the sinus endoscope.**

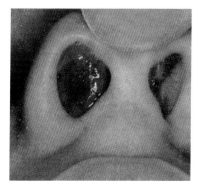

Fig. 3.**88 Nasal polyp extruding through the anterior nares.** Large nasal polyps prolapse into the nasal vestibule with the exposed surface losing the opalescent gray color.

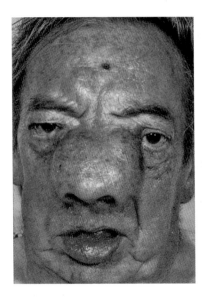

Fig. 3.**89 Extensive nasal polyps** may expand into the nasal bones, and the external deformity of the polyps may become gross. Surgical removal of the polyps may suffice in the elderly, in whom this complication is usually seen.

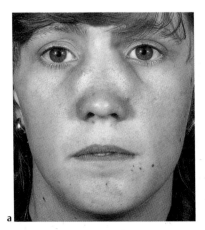

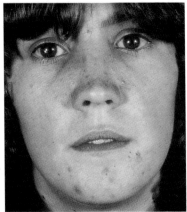

a   b

Fig. 3.**90a, b Nasal bone expansion** due to extensive nasal polyps in the younger patient (**a**) also requires rhinoplasty to restore appearance (**b**).

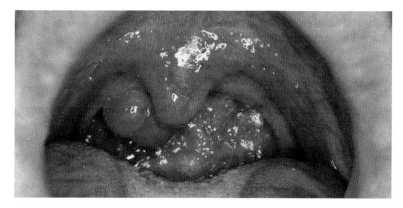

Fig. 3.**91 Nasal polyps in the oropharynx.** Extensive nasal polyps may extend beyond the soft palate and present in the oropharynx.

Antrochoanal Polyp and Angiofibroma

This is a special type of nasal polyp occurring in adolescents and young adults. Unilateral nasal obstruction is caused by a gray single polyp seen in the postnasal space. The maxillary sinus is opaque on radiograph.

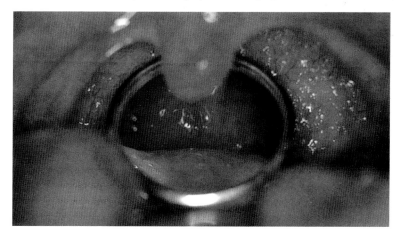

Fig. 3.**92 Antrochoanal polyp** seen with the postnasal mirror. A large antrochoanal polyp may present below the soft palate. A solitary polyp in one choana is almost certainly an antrochoanal polyp, but a vascular polyp that should be remembered as a differential diagnosis is the *angiofibroma of male puberty.*

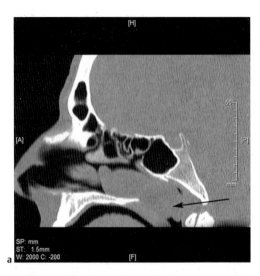

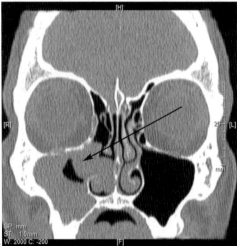

Fig. 3.**93a, b Antrochoanal polyp.** The dumbbell-shaped polyp extrudes through the widened ostium (arrow in **a**) to prolapse into the postnasal space (arrow in **b**).

Fig. 3.**94a, b The angiofibroma of male puberty** is a rare vascular malformation in the ▶ postnasal space, which may become extremely large, presenting with nasal obstruction and epistaxis. Treatment is difficult, but surgical removal via a midfacial "degloving" approach (**a, b**) allows access via the midfacial skeleton without facial scars. Some facial fractures and other midfacial tumors can be managed via this approach. Very large angiofibroma being removed from the postnasal space.

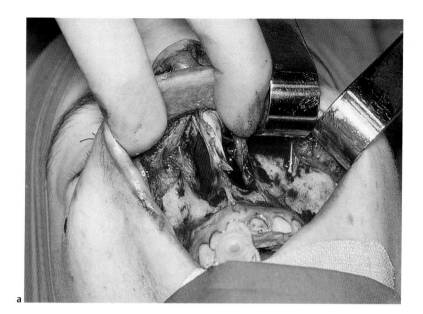

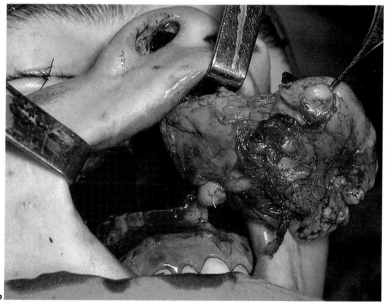

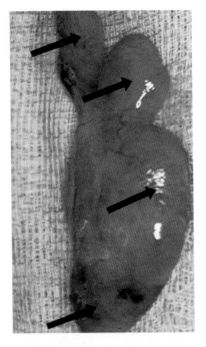

Fig. 3.**95 Antrochoanal polyp.** This type of polyp, which arises from the antral mucosa, extrudes through the ostium to fill the posterior nasal fossa and postnasal space. It frequently becomes extremely large and extends below the soft palate. Removal of the polyp from its origin in the antrum endoscopically or via a sublabial antrostomy approach may be necessary (Fig 3.**85**).

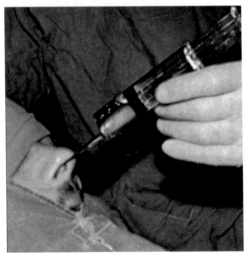

Fig. 3.**96 Aspiration from the antrum.** This shows straw-colored fluid, and is a reliable diagnostic test for an antrochoanal polyp.

Fungal Sinusitis

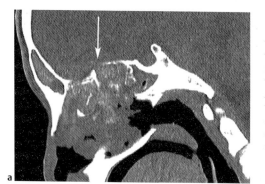

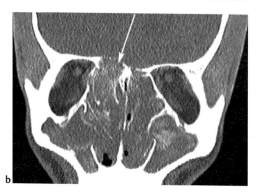

Fig. 3.**97a, b Fungal sinusitis.** Fungal infections take various forms. This allergic form of fungal sinusitis has caused expansion and erosion of bone of the anterior skull base (arrows). An endoscopic approach via the nose is usually used, but an external surgical cranio-facial approach may be necessary (see p. 165)

Epistaxis

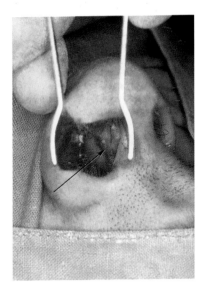

Fig. 3.98 Epistaxis. Anteriorly on the septum there is anastomosis of several arteries (the sphenopalatine, the greater palatine, the superior labial, and the anterior ethmoidal). This site is called Little's area or Kiesselbach's plexus, and is the commonest site of nose bleeds. Although associated with alarm, most epistaxis is short-lived and trivial. It is better to sit upright since the blood tends to be swallowed, causing nausea on lying down. There are numerous causes of epistaxis. Some, such as trauma and acute inflammatory nasal conditions, are obvious and common, but the more serious local and general causes must not be overlooked. Diagnosis must follow control of the epistaxis. Hypertension and blood dyscrasia are important general causes; neoplasms and teleangiectasia may also be underlying local factors.

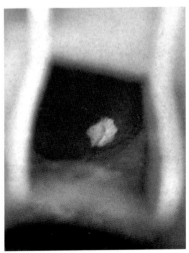

Fig. 3.99 Cautery. If epistaxis is recurrent, cautery (which is painless with local anesthetic) to the bleeding point is necessary, either with galvanocautery or with a chemical (e. g., trichloracetic acid or silver nitrate). Trichloracetic acid used in this case causes the bleeding site in Little's area to become white.

Care must be taken to avoid the chemicals running onto the skin of the vestibule or face, as scarring will result. A topical anesthetic is applied to the nasal mucous membrane in Little's area for galvanocautery but, with silver nitrate and trichloracetic acid, no anesthetic is needed, and the procedure is painless providing the vestibular skin is not touched.

It may be preferable for cautery to be carried out with the patient lying down, and with the help of the operating microscope (see Fig. 1.**15a**).

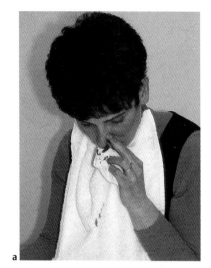
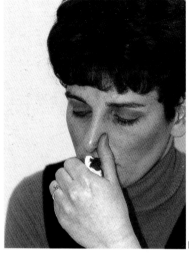

a   b

Fig. 3.**100a, b Control of epistaxis.** Firm pressure with the finger or thumb on the lateral wall of the nose opposite Little's area on the side of the bleeding, if maintained for about four minutes, will control the bleeding.

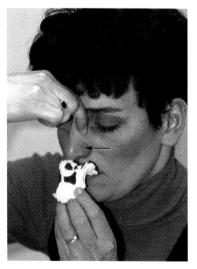

Fig. 3.**101 Incorrect technique for controlling epistaxis.** The pressure is over the nasal bones and ineffective. The arrow indicates the site where pressure should be applied.

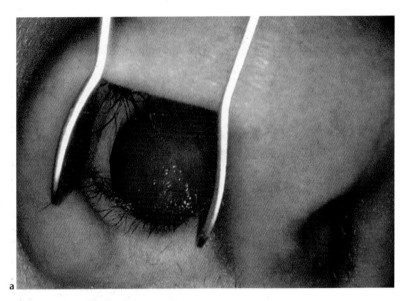

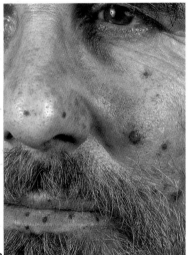

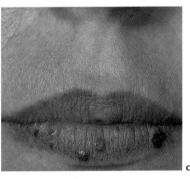

Fig. 3.**102a–f Hereditary nasal teleangiectasia.** Frequent and often severe epistaxis is characteristic of this condition, in which numerous leashes of bleeding vessels are apparent over the nasal mucosa (**a**). Telangiectasia are also seen elsewhere in the body—on the skin of the cheek (**b**), the lips (**c**), the tongue (**d**), the hands (**e**) and fingernails (**f**).   Fig. 3.**102d–f** ▶

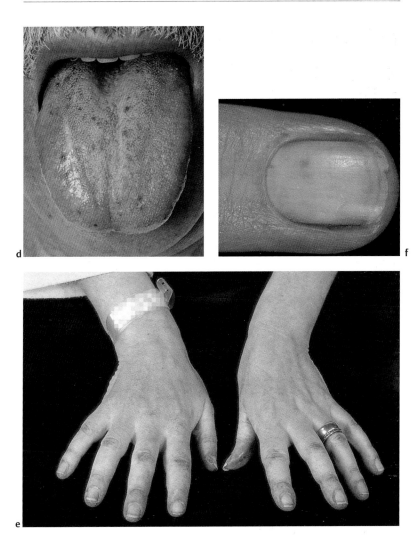

Fig. 3.**102a–f** (cont.) Cautery may be effective in the early stages, but this condition is difficult to manage, and may require either extensive skin grafting of the nasal septum to replace the vascular septal mucosa, or estrogen therapy.

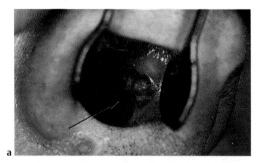

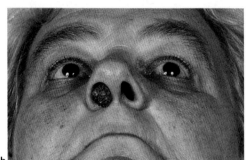

Fig. 3.**103a, b Septal hemangioma. a** A vascular sessile polyp is seen on the septum (hemangioma), which is the cause of severe, recurrent bleeds. Treatment is by excision, or cautery if the lesion is small.

b A *large septal hemangioma* occluding the nasal vestibule. Sometimes this is called a "bleeding polypus of the septum." Nasal hemangiomas may develop during pregnancy and be a cause of epistaxis at this time.

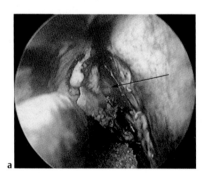

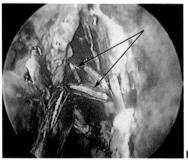

Fig. 3.**104a, b Endoscopic sphenopalatine artery ligation** with titanium clips may be the surgical procedure necessary for severe epistaxis. Single arrow shows the sphenopalatine artery; the double arrows show the clips ligating the arteries.

Epistaxis from the anterior septum may be profuse and alarming, but firm sustained pressure on the nares is invariably effective. Posterior epistaxis from the sphenopalatine artery may be very severe and difficult to manage. Nasal packing is needed to control the acute phase.

A posterior bleeding site may be identified with the nasal endoscope and cauterized. With more severe bleeding, ligation techniques are used. Success is greater when vessels close to the likely bleeding point are ligated (Fig. 3.**104a,b**).

The terminal branch of the anterior ethmoidal artery may be the site of bleeding superiorly in the nose, particularly with nasal fractures; this vessel may require ligation. Radiographic techniques enable embolism of the terminal vessels to be carried out via an arterial catheter, and this is an option in managing very severe epistaxis, which may become life threatening. However, there is a higher rate of embolic and ischemic complications.

Neoplasms

A nasal polyp that does not appear gray and opalescent should arouse suspicion, as should a polyp that bleeds spontaneously. A solid-looking hyperemic polyp may be an **inverted papilloma**. Granulation tissue in the nose may be malignant granuloma or carcinoma, and biopsy of any suspicious nasal lesion is necessary.

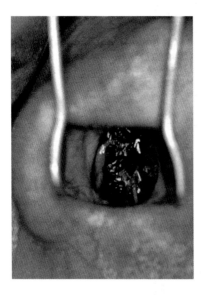

Fig. 3.**105 A pigmented polyp** may be a malignant melanoma.

Prognosis when radiotherapy is followed by maxillectomy is quite good for an early maxillary carcinoma, but poor when there is extensive invasion. Exenteration of the orbit with maxillectomy is necessary when the base of the skull is involved. The use of cytotoxic drugs results in regression in some of these paranasal sinus neoplasms and is a further line of treatment. Extension of a neoplasm superiorly into the anterior cranial fossa involves resection superiorly of the dura and involved frontal lobe of the brain in continuity with the nasal and sinus neoplasms (**cranio-facial resection**).

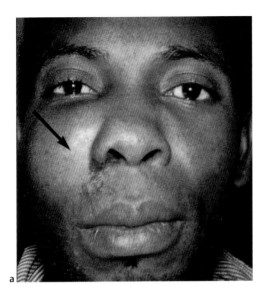

Fig. 3.**106a, b Carcinoma of the antrum or ethmoid.** These may extend not only into the nasal fossa and cheek (**a**, arrow), but may present in the oral cavity (**b**, arrow), appearing as a dental lesion.

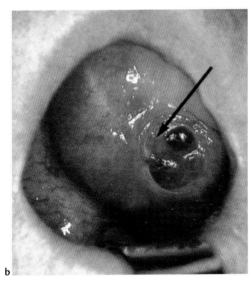

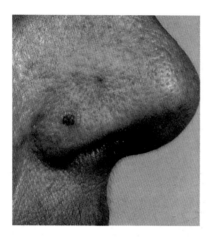

Fig. 3.**107 Basal cell carcinoma of the nose.** One should be suspicious of an apparently innocent but chronic skin lesion (arrow) which slowly increases in size and may bleed. Excision with a good margin is curative (see p. 177). If, however, these lesions are ignored—and frequently they are disguised with cosmetics for months and even years—their excision can present considerable problems of reconstruction to avoid deformity in such an obvious site as the region of the nasal tip.

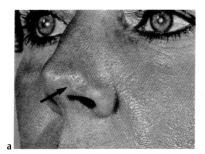

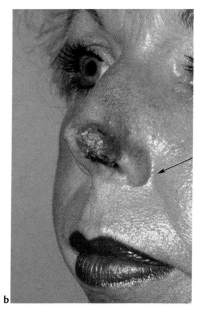

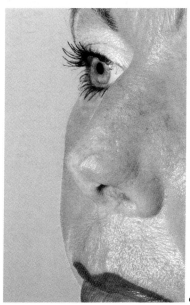

Fig. 3.**108a–c Repair following excision of nasal tip basal cell carcinoma.** A large defect may remain in an obvious site (**a**, arrow). In this instance, a composite graft (a graft of two or three tissue layers) taken from the cartilage and skin of the ear was used as a free graft to repair the nasal tip (**c**).

The composite ear graft takes time to vascularize and the appearance of the graft in the early days may not look promising (**b**).

Basal cell carcinomas in the groove at the base of the alae tend to erode deeply (**b**, arrow). Radiotherapy is the alternative treatment to surgery, and with modern super-voltage therapy, lesions overlying cartilages can be treated with minimal risk of perichondritis.

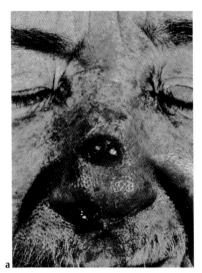 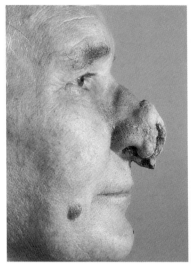

a   b

Fig. 3.**109a, b Carcinoma of the nose. a** The apex of the nasal vestibule must be examined extremely carefully in a case of scanty epistaxis, where no obvious bleeding site is apparent in Little's area.

Minimal bleeding and occasional serosanguineous discharge were this patient's presenting complaints.

Later, the carcinoma became obvious, having eroded through the skin of the dorsum of the nose.

b Wide surgical excision with forehead reconstruction rhinoplasty or, less commonly, radiotherapy, are the available treatments.

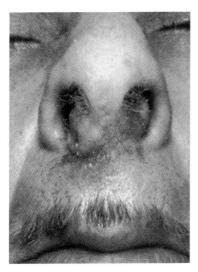

Fig. 3.**110 Carcinoma of the septum and columella.**

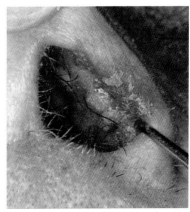

Fig. 3.**111 Squamous cell carcinoma of the nasal vestibule.** The history was short, and the differential diagnosis of a basal cell carcinoma was made at biopsy.

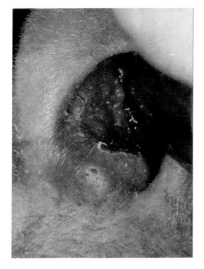

Fig. 3.**112 Carcinoma of the nasal septum.** A biopsy of this ulcer on the septum and columella, which presented with scanty epistaxis, confirmed squamous cell carcinoma.

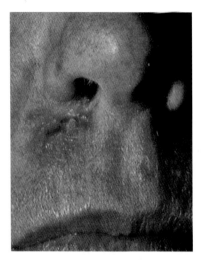

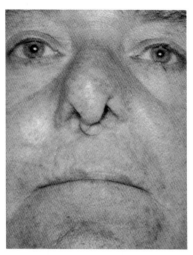

Fig. 3.**113 Chronic inflammation of the nose.** Lupus vulgaris is now rare. It presents as a chronic ulcer of the nasal vestibule extending onto the face. The differential diagnosis of inflammatory ulceration anteriorly in the nose includes sarcoidosis, which may also cause destruction of the ala. Biopsy is necessary for the diagnosis.

Fig. 3.**114 The effects of lupus vulgaris.** Lupus, if ignored, is destructive to the skin and cartilage of the alae nasi and septum.

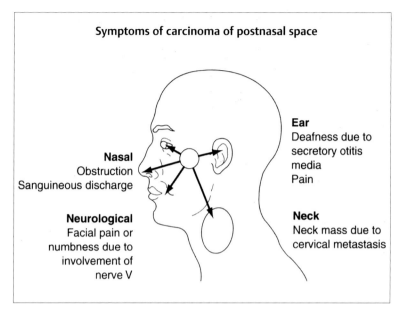

Symptoms of carcinoma of postnasal space

Ear
Deafness due to secretory otitis media
Pain

Nasal
Obstruction
Sanguineous discharge

Neurological
Facial pain or numbness due to involvement of nerve V

Neck
Neck mass due to cervical metastasis

Fig. 3.**115 Symptoms of carcinoma of postnasal space.** This is uncommon in most countries, but has an unexplained high incidence in the Far East (particularly China) and East Africa. There are many presenting symptoms. As the posterior choanae are large, nasal obstruction is not common with ulcerated carcinomas, which tend to present with symptoms of nerve involvement or otitis media with effusion due to interference with the eustachian tube. Lymphosarcomas and papilliferous carcinomas, however, cause obstruction. Carcinoma invades the skull base, involving nerves V, VI, and the Vidian (pterygoid) nerve, and may cause headache by invasion of the dura. The nasopharynx is a relatively concealed site, and presentation of carcinoma is commonly late, with a cervical node metastasis. The treatment is with radiotherapy. The overall prognosis is not good, with about a 30% five-year survival rate. This is, however, mainly related to the late diagnosis. An awareness of the early presenting symptoms and signs is essential for improved prognosis.

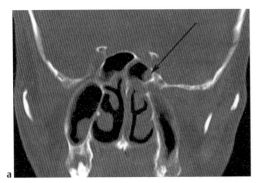

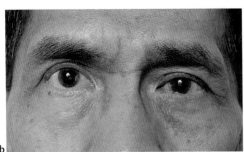

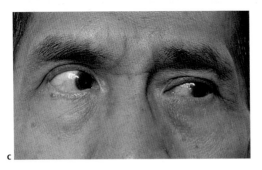

Fig. 3.**116 a Direct extension of carcinoma through the skull base**, as shown on this CT scan (arrow).

b, c Local spread of the tumor through the skull base has resulted in a left cranial nerve VI palsy causing diplopia when the patient looks to the left as shown.

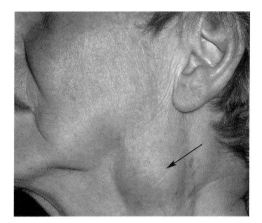

Fig. 3.**117 Carcinoma of the postnasal space**, presenting with a metastatic cervical lymph node (arrow).

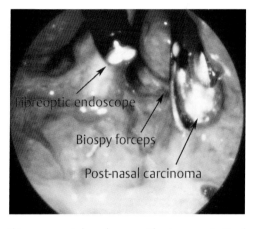

Fig. 3.**118 Carcinoma of the postnasal space.** A photograph through the fiberoptic endoscope gives a clear view of this postnasal space carcinoma.

The biopsy forceps also introduced through the anterior nares can be seen. Therefore, biopsy of a postnasal carcinoma can be carried out as an outpatient procedure under local anesthetic, using the fiberoptic endoscope.

Prior to the introduction of this instrument, the postnasal space was a "hidden" site, as this area cannot always be seen with mirror examination (see Fig. 1.**47a**). General anesthesia was necessary for a thorough examination and biopsy.

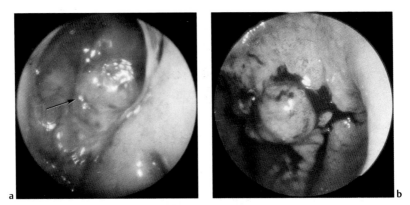

a

b

Fig. 3.**119a, b Carcinoma of the postnasal space** (**a**, arrow) seen well with the endoscope adjacent to the eustachian cushion. Some bleeding shows the site of a biopsy of the postnasal carcinoma taken via the endoscope (**b**).

4 The Pharynx and Larynx

The Oropharynx, Mouth, and Lips

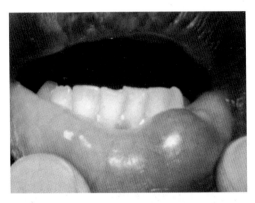

Fig. 4.1 **A mucocele of the lip.** Mucoceles are cystic, non-tender swellings presenting on the lips or in the oral cavity. They result from extravasation of mucus from a mucous gland into the surrounding tissue. Treatment is excision, which is not always easy because of the extremely thin wall. Simple marsupialization is often adequate.

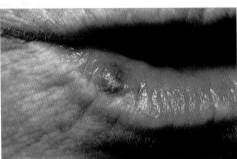

Fig. 4.2 **A hemangioma of the lip.** These may require excision or laser surgery from a cosmetic point of view or on account of bleeding with trauma.

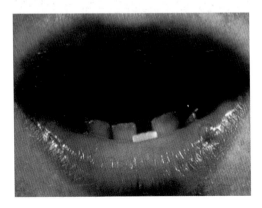

Fig. 4.3 **Lip ulcers.** Lip ulceration has numerous causes, either traumatic, inflammatory, or neoplastic. The provisional diagnosis can be made from the history and type of ulcer. Biopsy is necessary to confirm the diagnosis. This lesion is a *pyogenic granuloma*. Although these lesions are frequently small and related to trauma, they may enlarge from secondary infection (see Fig. 4.4) and take several weeks to heal.

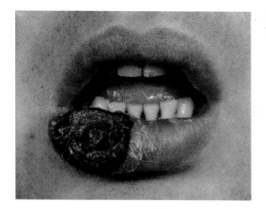

Fig. 4.**4** **Lip ulcer enlarging from secondary infection.**

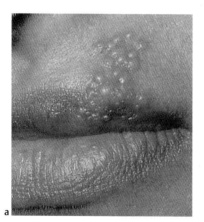

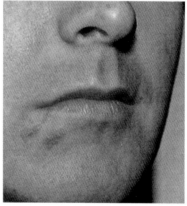

a

b

Fig. 4.**5a, b Herpes simplex of the lip** showing the characteristic vesicles (**a**) which later crust (**b**).

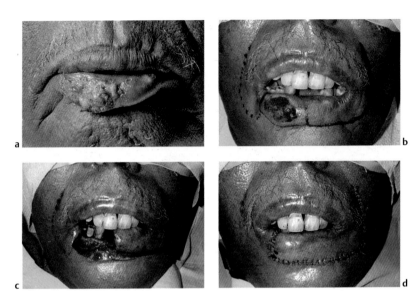

Fig. 4.**6a–d Carcinoma of the lower lip**. A biopsy is taken from the lesion margin. Excision with wide margin is outlined. Large rotational flaps are necessary to close the resulting defect.

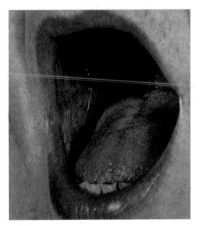

Fig. 4.**7 Keratosis** may extend from the angle of the mouth along the occlusal plane of the teeth and is commonly a dental problem; it may be self-induced due to nervous cheek-biting. It is often the result of persistent trauma to the mucous membrane.

When occurring in a site not exposed to trauma, e. g., the retromolar fossa, it should arouse suspicion that the mucosal change may be malignant and, therefore, a biopsy is necessary.

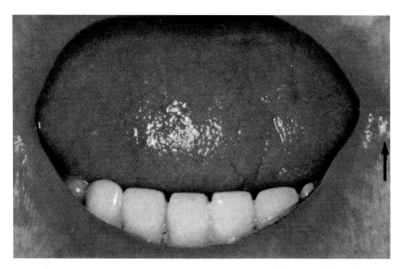

Fig. 4.**8 Angular stomatitis** (arrow) occurs with the type of dental hyperkeratosis shown in Fig. 4.**7**, but it may also be part of the Plummer–Vinson or Patterson–Brown–Kelly syndromes in which glossitis (also seen here) and hypochromic anemia are associated with a postcricoid lesion, either a web or a carcinoma. This syndrome occurs mostly in women.

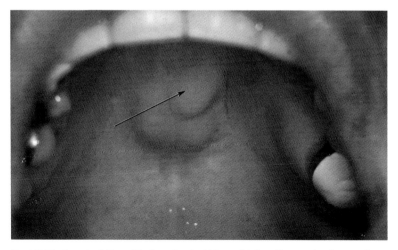

Fig. 4.**9 The torus palatinus.** The bony hard mid-line palatal swelling can be diagnosed confidently by these characteristics (arrow). It is a common finding, and only requires removal if it interferes with the fitting of a denture.

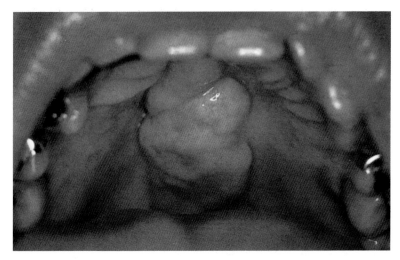

Fig. 4.**10 A large torus palatinus** may take on a curious, irregular appearance suspicious of a carcinoma. Similar bony swellings occur on the lingual surface of the lower alveolus opposite the premolars (torus mandibularis).

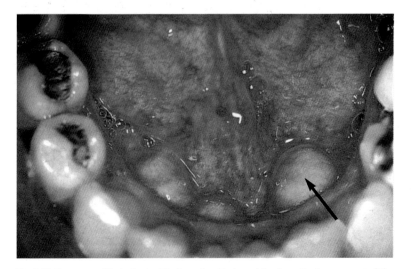

Fig. 4.**11 Torus mandibularis.** A white bony hard lesion arising from the inner aspect of the mandible may present as a swelling in the floor of the mouth (arrow). This is considerably less common than the torus palatinus.

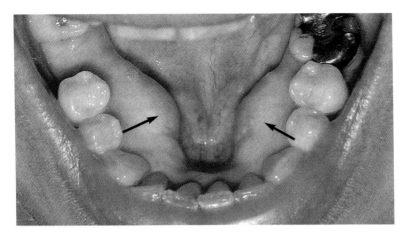

Fig. 4.**12 A bilateral torus mandibularis (arrows).**

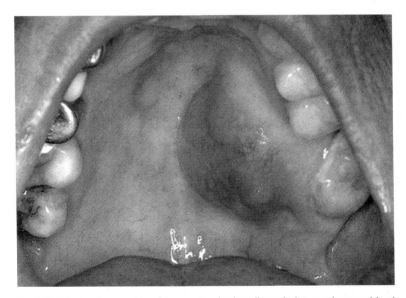

Fig. 4.**13 Ectopic pleomorphic adenoma.** A palatal swelling which is not bony and hard may be a fissural cyst if mid-line, but if placed to one side (as it is here), it is almost certainly a tumor of one of the minor salivary glands. Biopsy is necessary. It is frequently a pleomorphic adenoma, but may be an adenoid cystic carcinoma or other malignant salivary tumor. A tumor extension from the maxillary antrum must also be excluded.

Aphthous Ulcers

An area of white superficial ulceration is surrounded by a hyperemic mucous membrane. These commonly occur in crops of two or more, and heal spontaneously in about one week. They are also acutely tender, and affect the nonkeratinized oral mucous membrane. Although there is no induration on palpation, the histological inflammatory changes are not superficial, and may extend into the underlying muscle.

Hydrocortisone pellets to suck, or triamcinolone with Orabase ointments applied to the ulcer, are the most effective present treatments to relieve the pain. As the etiology of these extremely common ulcers remains unknown, treatment is empirical.

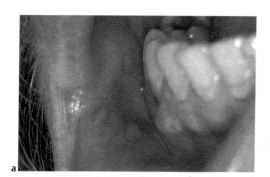

Fig. 4.**14a, b Aphthous ulcers.**

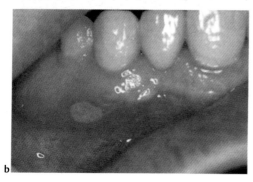

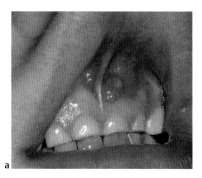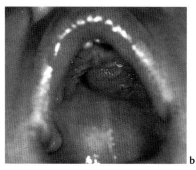

a   b

Fig. 4.**15a, b Ulceration and swelling of dental origin. a** An aphthous-like ulcer overlying the apex of this deciduous tooth suggests the diagnosis of an apical dental abscess. **b** A palatal abscess of dental origin.

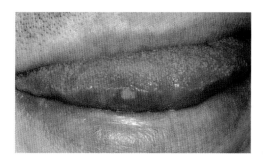

Fig. 4.**16 Aphthous ulcers on the tongue.** Aphthous ulcers on the tongue margin are often traumatic from tooth irregularity.

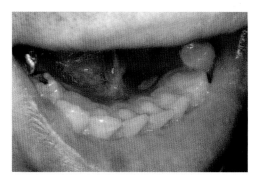

Fig. 4.**17 Trauma from a denture.** This may be an irritating factor, as may any minor trauma to the mucous membrane in a person susceptible to aphthous ulcers.

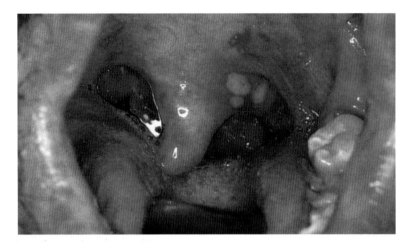

Fig. 4.**18 Aphthous ulcers on the soft palate.** Aphthous ulcers are not uncommon on the soft palate.

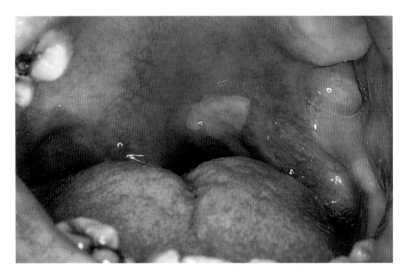

Fig. 4.**19 Solitary aphthous ulcer.** This ulcer (*periadenitis mucosa necrotica recurrens*) looks similar to a simple aphthous ulcer and is the same histologically, but it behaves differently. It is less common, larger, persists for several weeks or months and may leave a scar. It occurs in more varied sites affecting the soft palate and even the pyriform fossa, where it presents with severe dysphagia. Carbenoxolone is used topically for the lesions in the oral cavity.

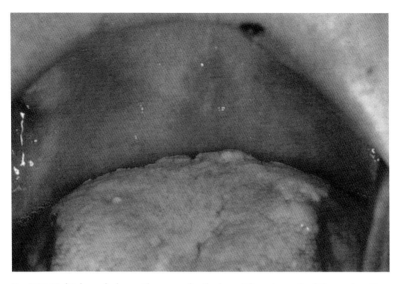

Fig. 4.**20 Multiple oral ulcers.** These may be the herpetiform type of aphthous ulceration, but are possibly caused by a blood dyscrasia. If the ulcers are crusted and hemorrhagic, the condition is either ***erythema multiforme*** or ***pemphigus***. Hemorrhagic bullae may also be seen on the soft and hard palate. An iritis and genital ulceration may be present (Behçet's syndrome). High doses of systemic steroids are usually needed to control this type of severe ulceration.

The snail-track ulcers of **secondary syphilis** must be remembered also in the differential diagnosis of oral ulceration (see Fig. 4.**62**).

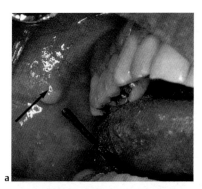

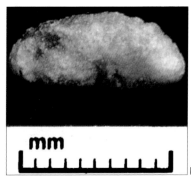

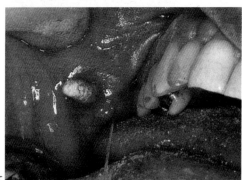

Fig. 4.**21a–c Parotid salivary calculus.** An ulcer in the region of the orifice of the parotid duct (**a,** arrow) suggests a possible salivary calculus. Parotid calculi are considerably less common than those in the sub-mandibular duct, but occasionally they may occlude the orifice of the duct, causing painful intermittent parotid swelling which requires incision and removal (**b, c**).

The Tongue

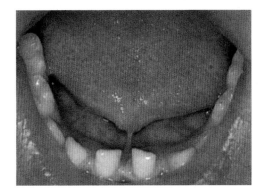

Fig. 4.**22** **"Tongue tie."** This is due to a short frenulum linguae, and apart from the defect of being unable to protrude the tongue, the patient is almost always symptom-free. Speech defects can rarely be attributed to tongue tie necessitating division of the frenulum.

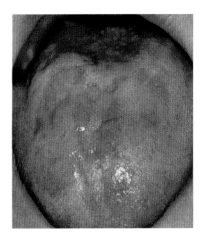

Fig. 4.**23** **Geographic tongue** (benign migratory glossitis). There are smooth areas with no filiform papillae. These areas vary in site on the tongue, and the appearance may concern the patient. It is, however, a condition of no significance requiring no treatment other than reassurance.

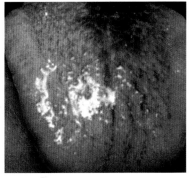

Fig. 4.**24** **Black hairy tongue.** Patients not infrequently regard the appearance of their tongue as an index of their general health, and are concerned upon seeing a brown-black staining. This may be fungal (*Aspergillus niger*) and related to prolonged antibiotic therapy, but is frequently a chance finding with no other pathology than hypertrophy of the filiform papillae. Tobacco may be a cause. Scraping and cleaning the tongue temporarily improves the appearance, but is unnecessary since this condition is harmless.

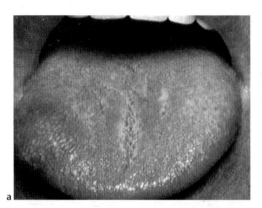

Fig. 4.**25a, b** **Hemangiomas of the tongue.** These may be chance findings and are usually innocuous. If large and giving rise to bleeding, laser surgery is the most effective present treatment.

a

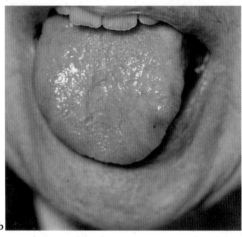

b

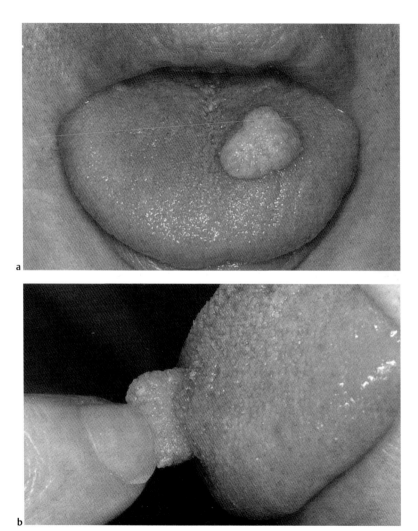

Fig. 4.**26a, b Papilloma of the tongue.** Benign lesions of the tongue are common, and are either sessile or pedunculated (**b**). Simple excision under local anesthetic with biopsy is required.

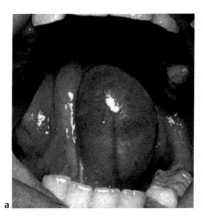

a

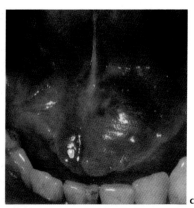

c

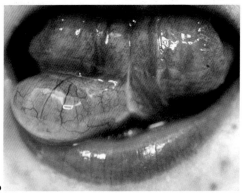

b

Fig. 4.**27a–c The ranula** is a mucocele occurring in the floor of the mouth (**a, b**). A blue color and the profunda vein stretched across the surface are characteristic. A ranula may extend into the tissues of the floor of the mouth and neck (plunging ranula). Total surgical removal is difficult because of the thin wall, and marsupialization is adequate treatment. Recurrence is not uncommon.

The ranula may also present more in the floor of the mouth than on the undersurface of the tongue, and the diagnosis may not be so obvious. **c** A less well-defined ranula occupying the floor of the mouth.

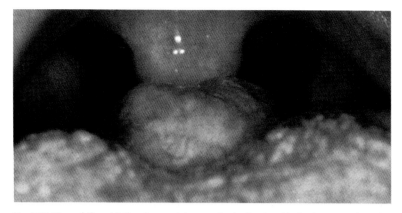

Fig. 4.**28 Lingual thyroid.** Developmental anomalies in the thyroid gland may result in thyroid tissue remaining at the foramen caecum or in the thyroglossal tract. The symptom-free swelling at the base of this tongue is thyroid tissue, and was shown on a radioactive iodine scan to be active. No thyroid gland was palpable in the neck, and there was no iodine uptake other than at the base of the tongue. This lingual thyroid, therefore, was this patient's only active thyroid tissue.

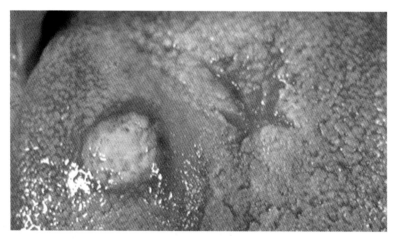

Fig. 4.**29 Tongue ulceration.** The site and type of tongue ulcers give the provisional diagnosis: A marginal ulcer with a raised edge is probably a carcinoma; an ulcer on the dorsum with a punched-out margin may be a gumma. Tuberculosis may be the cause of a tender ulcer on the tip of the tongue in an area where tuberculosis is prevalent. However, these clinical findings are only guides. Biopsy of this ulcer on the dorsum showed it to be a solitary aphthous ulcer (Fig. 4.**19**).

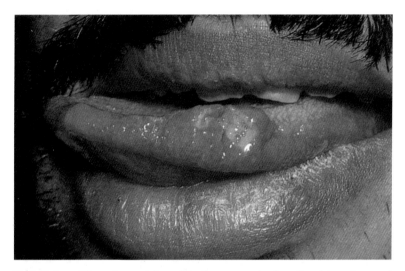

Fig. 4.**30 An aphthous tongue ulcer** of the tongue may be deceptive. A buccal mucosal aphthous ulcer is flat, but on the tongue some swelling due to trauma may make a biopsy necessary in order to be certain of the diagnosis.

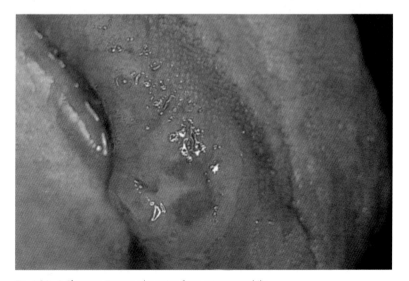

Fig. 4.**31 A Chancre.** Tongue ulceration from primary syphilis.

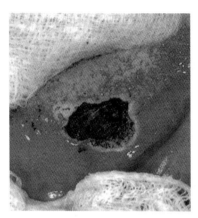

Fig. 4.**32 Laser excision of a tongue lesion.** This shows the minimal reaction at the excision margin, and the nonbleeding base of the excision.

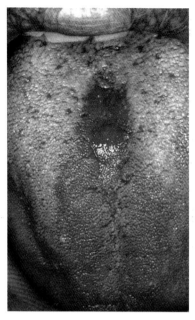

Fig. 4.**33 Median rhomboid glossitis.** This rare anomaly results from failure of the lateral halves of the tongue to fuse posteriorly, leaving the tuberculum impar in the midline. A smooth, red, usually symptom-free area persists.

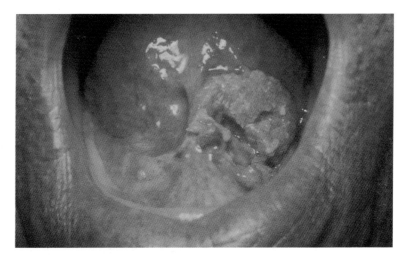

Fig. 4.**34 Carcinoma of the tongue.** This usually occurs on the margin or from the extension of an ulcer on the floor of the mouth (as shown here). Biopsy of this proliferative ulcer showed squamous cell carcinoma. Partial glossectomy in continuity with a neck dissection, or radiotherapy, are the current treatments.

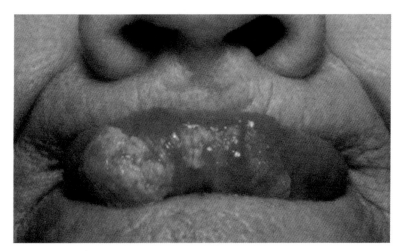

Fig. 4.**35 Leukoplakia.** This is precarcinomatous on the tongue. It may be secondary to dental or dietary irritation. Leukoplakia is also characteristic of tertiary syphilis, and the tongue is a site where the spirochaete predisposes to carcinoma. Leukoplakia, particularly with no apparent underlying traumatic cause, should be biopsied to exclude carcinoma.

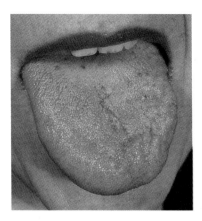

Fig. 4.**36 Hypoglossal nerve paralysis.** Initially, there is fibrillation and later atrophy of the muscles on one side of the tongue. The tongue deviates on protrusion to the side of the nerve palsy. A destructive lesion in the jugular foramen region may extend to involve the hypoglossal nerve as it emerges from the nearby anterior condylar foramen. This paralysis of the tongue shows wrinkling caused by fibrillation, and is due to a glomus jugulare tumor, which has also damaged the cranial nerves emerging through the jugular foramen (IX, X, and XI).

The hypoglossal nerve, if involved in cervical metastases, may be sectioned in a radical neck dissection (see p. 243).

The Fauces and the Tonsils

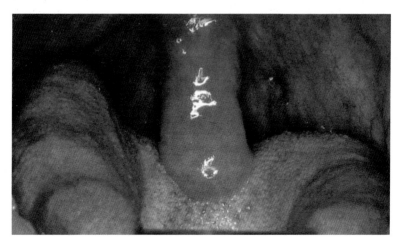

Fig. 4.**37 The uvula.** This obvious anatomical feature in the oropharynx has little pathological significance. When particularly long, however, as here, it has on occasion been thought responsible for various throat symptoms such as discomfort and snoring. Partial amputation has been recommended.

The uvula is excised along with part of the tonsillar fauces and soft palate in the operation of ***uvulopalatoplasty*** for snoring. The appearance of the palate after operation is seen in Figs. 4.**40b** and 4.**69**.

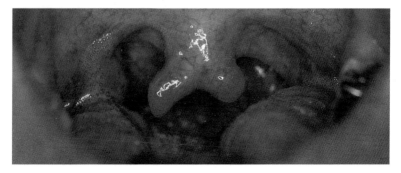

Fig. 4.**38 Bifid uvula.** A common minor congenital deformity of the palate.

It is of little significance, but it may be associated with a submucous palatal cleft. Inflammation of the uvula as an isolated entity may occur, however, and a cherry-like enlargement may be the sole presenting sign of a sore throat (uvulitis).

Snoring

Snoring, although in most cases a relatively trivial problem, may if gross have serious implications. Although snoring is commonly associated with obesity, aging, (where the pharyngeal tissues become more lax) along with late-night excess food and alcohol intake, there are anatomical factors in the upper respiratory tract that contribute to snoring. Nasal obstruction accentuates snoring but is not commonly the prime cause. Surgery therefore for airway problems to the nose may not be curative.

The anatomy of the soft palate and oropharynx however is a cause of snoring when the soft palate, uvula and fauces are long and lax. Large tonsils may also cause snoring. Surgery to reduce the size and mobility of the soft palate—uvulopalatoplasty—has become established world-wide. The uvula and soft palate are "stiffened" with diathermy, partial excision, radiofrequency surgery, or laser techniques. Short-term success rates are good but the snoring may recur.

Sleep nasendoscopy helps define whether the cause of snoring is in the oropharynx, tongue base, or nose. Sleep studies measure the respiratory rate, cardiac function, O_2, CO_2, and chest movement with video monitoring in sleep as shown (Fig. 4.**39**).

Sleep studies are carried out preoperatively for assessment of the snoring. Apart from appraising the predominant site causing the snoring, whether the oropharynx, tongue base, or nose, sleep studies monitor the respiration rate, cardiac function with O_2 and CO_2 levels during sleep.

With gross snoring both in children (where upper respiratory tract obstruction from marked adenoids and tonsil hypertrophy may be relevant) and in adults, significant physiological upset may ensure. With **sleep apnea** respiration is sufficiently disturbed by snoring to cause cardiac arrhythmia and maybe cardiac enlargement, along with periods of oxygen deficit.

In these instances treatment for snoring either by surgery or by oxygen administration at night is necessary along with other steps, for example, weight loss. Mandibular advancement splints (MAS) (Fig. 4.**41**) have become an important nonsurgical treatment which increases the dimensions of the upper airway, improving both snoring and obstructive sleep apnea syndrome. Oxygen supplied at night prevents sleep apnea—continuous positive airway pressure (CPAP; Fig. 4.**40c**). A mask is firmly attached to the nose to supply oxygen; the patient's discomfort may limit the application of this treatment.

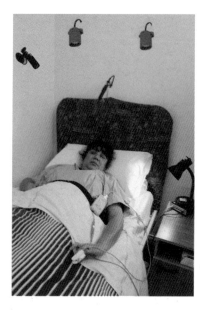

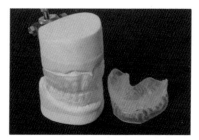

Fig. 4.**41 Mandibular advancement splints** (MAS) pull forward the bulky tongue base.

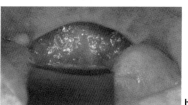

◄ **Fig. 4.39   Multiple-channel sleep studies** record heart rate, oxygen saturation, and chest movements.

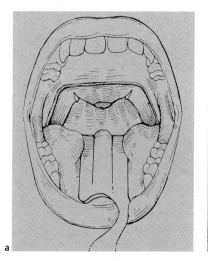

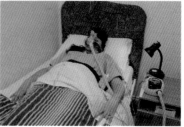

Fig. 4.**40a–c Snoring. a, b** Uvuloplasty to remove the uvula and shorten the faucial pillars. **c** An oxygen mask may be worn at night to prevent sleep apnea.

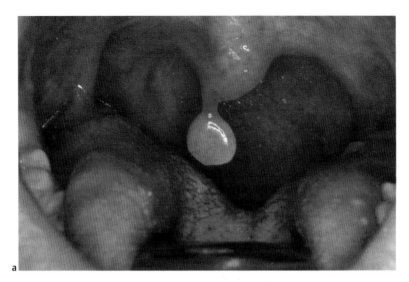

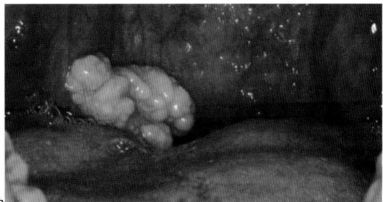

Fig. 4.**42a, b Papillomas.** These may occur on the uvula (**a**), fauces, and tonsil. The patient often notices these papillomas when looking at the throat, or they are found at medical examination. Symptoms are uncommon. They are usually pedunculated and are easily and painlessly removable in outpatients. They should be sent for histology to exclude a squamous carcinoma. If ignored, a papilloma may cause symptoms on account of size. This large papilloma (**b**) arises from the base of the right tonsil.

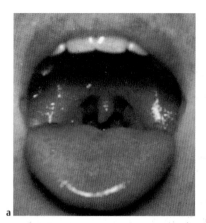
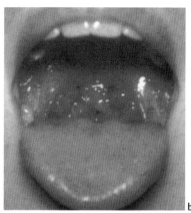

a   b

Fig. 4.**43a, b Tonsil size.** There is no recognized "normal" size for a tonsil. It is, therefore, arguable as to whether tonsils can be described as "enlarged." The apparent size of the tonsil can be altered considerably when the tongue is protruded forcibly. This child, whose oropharynx looks normal when the tongue is slightly protruded (**a**), can make the tonsils meet in the mid-line with maximum protrusion of the tongue (**b**).

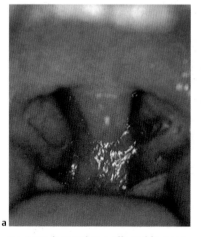
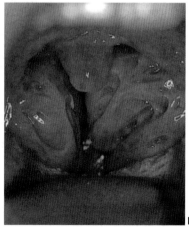

a   b

Fig. 4.**44a, b Tonsil size affected by tongue depressor.** The tongue depressor also alters the apparent size of the tonsils. If the tongue is firmly depressed, the patient gags and the tonsils meet in the mid-line (**b**).

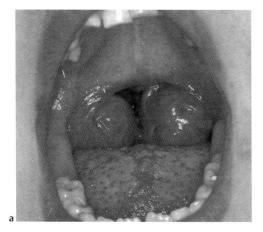

a

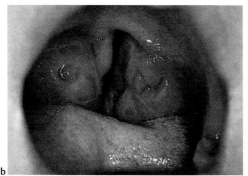

b

Fig. 4.**45a, b Tonsils meeting in the mid-line.** It is unusual for tonsils to meet in the midline or to overlap. Lymphoid tissue of this bulk, particularly during an acute tonsillitis, may cause respiratory obstruction and severe dysphagia. There is an increased awareness of the severity of upper respiratory tract obstruction from the bulk of tonsillar and adenoid lymphoid tissue.

In children, particularly at times of superimposed tonsillitis, the interference with breathing becomes alarming, and obstructive sleep apnea syndrome is now well-recognized as an important indication for surgery to remove the tonsils and adenoids. Cor pulmonale is seen in children with marked upper respiratory tract obstruction.

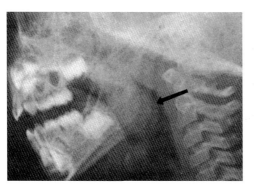

Fig. 4.**46 Lateral radiograph of tonsils.** The tonsils (arrow) and adenoids shown on lateral radiograph, and the soft-tissue shadow helps in assessing the degree of obstruction that the lymphoid tissue may be causing. The lingual tonsil is unusually large in Down's syndrome patients and contributes to their characteristic bulky tongue.

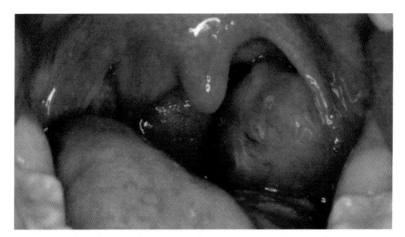

Fig. 4.**47 Unilateral tonsil enlargement.** A tonsil can be described as "large" when compared with the other tonsil. A conspicuously large tonsil in the absence of acute inflammation is an important finding suggesting either a ***chronic quinsy* or a *lymphosarcoma***. A persistent and conspicuously large tonsil, therefore, should be removed for histology.

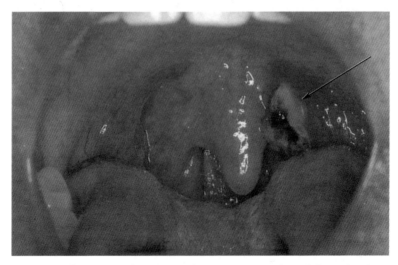

Fig. 4.**48 A palate and tonsil carcinoma.** This presents as an indurated ulcer rather than a diffuse enlargement, and causes referred ear pain. The biopsy is taken from the ulcer margin (arrow).

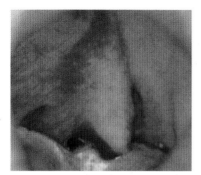

Fig. 4.**49 Simulated tonsil enlargement.** A tonsil may appear to be enlarged by medial displacement from a parapharyngeal swelling, and careful examination of the fauces ensures that the correct diagnosis is made. It is possible to biopsy a normal tonsil and realize later that medial displacement is simulating enlargement. In this case, the parapharyngeal mass is an internal carotid aneurysm. This initial diagnosis in Casualty was a quinsy—a dangerous error if followed by incision.

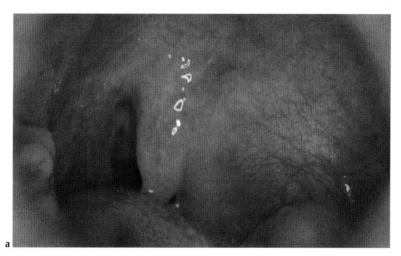

a

Fig. 4.**50a, b Tumors of the deep lobe of the parotid gland** may cause medial displacement of the tonsil. This appearance is also caused by less common parapharyngeal swellings, e.g., chemodectomas, neurofibromata, and enlargement of the parapharyngeal lymph nodes. **a** Clinical picture.

Fig. 4.**50b** ▶

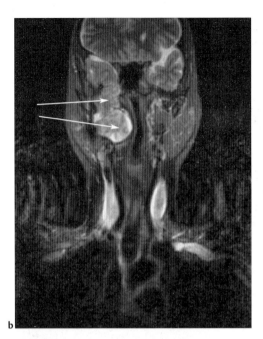

Fig. 4.**50b** MR image. The lobulated tumor seen (arrows) arises from the deep lobe of the parotid compressing the pharynx.

b

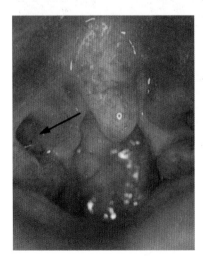

Fig. 4.**51 Supratonsillar cleft.** This recess near the superior pole of the tonsil, if large, tends to collect debris. A mass of yellow fetid material can be extruded from the tonsil with pressure; discomfort or halitosis are symptoms with which this condition may present. Tonsillectomy may be necessary. The surgeon, however, must beware of tonsillectomy for halitosis.

Although dental or gastric pathology may cause this symptom (as may a pharyngeal pouch), the symptom may be imagined by the patient, or by another person complaining about the halitosis.

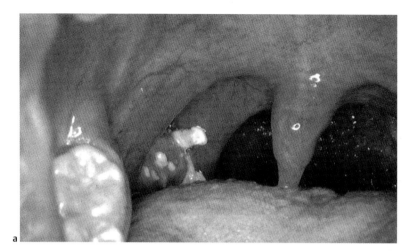

a

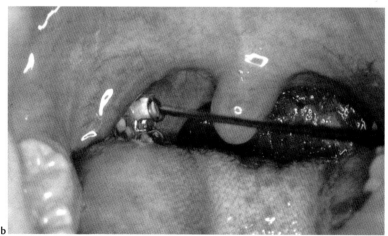

b

Fig. 4.**52a, b Keratosis pharyngeus.** Yellow spicules due to hyperkeratinized areas of epithelium are sometimes extensive over the tonsil and lingual tonsil (**a**). It is usually a chance finding, and it is important in diagnosis to probe the tonsil (**b**) to be certain that these yellow areas are not exudate. No treatment is required for this condition unless it is associated with tonsillitis.

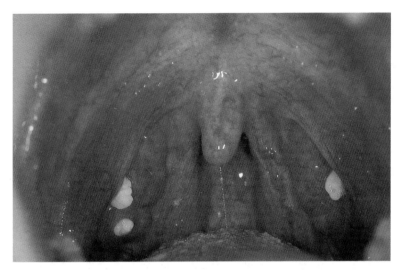

Fig. 4.**53 Tonsillar exudate.** Exudate from tonsillar crypts may appear indistinguishable from keratosis pharyngeus, and hence palpation with a probe is necessary.

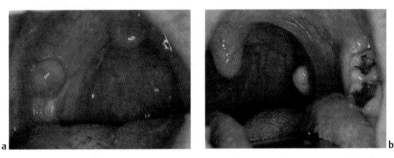

Fig. 4.**54a, b Retention cysts.** These are common on the tonsil and appear as sessile yellow swellings (**a**). If small they can be ignored, and although symptoms are uncommon, a concern by the patient or a sensation of a lump in the throat may call for surgical removal. Retention cysts are also seen following tonsillectomy in the region of the fauces (**b**).

Infections of the Tonsils, Pharynx, and Oropharynx

Acute Tonsillitis

This condition is characterized by sore throat, dysphagia, and pyrexia. The appearance of the tonsils varies. An obviously purulent exudate covering the tonsils is common, and is either diffuse or punctate (Fig. 4.**55a,b**). An apparently less severely infected throat with hyperemia of the tonsils only may, however, be associated with severe symptoms. The tonsillar lymph nodes near the angle of the mandible are large and tender.

With acute tonsillitis, the exudate and hyperemia are centered on the tonsils. In an acute pharyngitis, as may be associated with a head cold, the mucous membrane of the entire oropharynx is hyperemic.

The **gonococcus** may cause acute pharyngitis, and a throat swab must be placed in Stewart's medium for laboratory examination if this infection is suspected. The throat swab in acute tonsillitis commonly grows the **hemolytic streptococcus**, and a course of oral penicillin (often supplemented with an intramuscular injection) is invariably curative. An analgesic may also be needed, but lozenges and gargles are usually unnecessary.

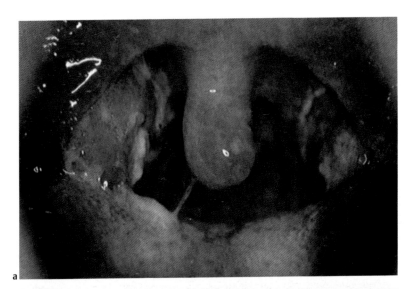

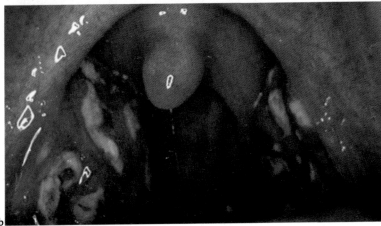

Fig. 4.**55a, b Acute tonsillitis.** The appearance of the tonsils in acute tonsillitis is either diffuse (**a**) or punctate (**b**).

Quinsy

This is a complication of acute tonsillitis in which a peritonsillar abscess forms. The symptoms may be extremely severe, with absolute dysphagia and pain referred to the ear and trismus, as well as malaise, fever, and marked swelling of the tonsillar lymph node. Examination shows the signs of acute tonsillitis with medial displacement of the tonsils to the mid-line.

If the abscess is pointing, incision at the site marked (Fig. 4.**56a,b**; arrows) releases the pus. Since the advent of antibiotics, there is less need for incision of quinsies. High doses of intramuscular penicillin for five days followed by a further five-day course of oral penicillin is the treatment. A large tonsil with medial displacement will persist with inadequate treatment, representing a chronic quinsy in which recurrence of an acute episode is common. A throat swab of the pus is taken at the time of diagnosis, and the result may later require changing the penicillin to another antibiotic.

A quinsy is extremely rare in children and is also rarely bilateral. Complications are uncommon, but bleeding from a quinsy is an important and serious sign: It is due to erosion by the peritonsillar pus of one of the adjacent vessels —either one of the tonsillar arteries or the internal carotid artery (***bleeding quinsy***).

Quinsies not infrequently occur in those who have suffered previous episodes of tonsillitis. Tonsillectomy, which is often indicated after a quinsy, is delayed by four to six weeks until the acute phase has passed. Vascular fibrous tissue found lateral to the tonsil after a quinsy make tonsillectomy technically difficult, and some advocate tonsillectomy at the time of the acute quinsy (***quinsy tonsillectomy***).

The pain with a quinsy is frequently so severe that swallowing is almost impossible and oral antibiotics cannot be given. Intravenous antibiotics, for example, penicillin supplemented with metronidazole (for there is a high instance of anaerobic organisms on culture) are given intravenously and usually bring about resolution in 24–48 hours.

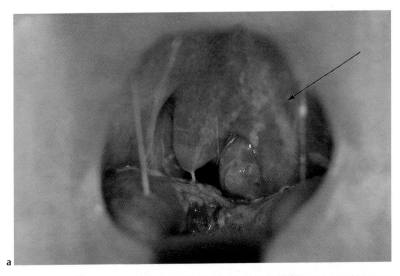

a

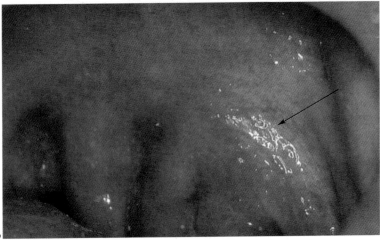

b

Fig. 4.**56a, b   Quinsy.**

Infectious Mononucleosis

Infectious mononucleosis should be suspected if a sore throat and malaise persist despite antibiotic treatment, or when a white membrane is apparent over the tonsil or pharynx. One should palpate for liver and spleen enlargement (hepatosplenomegaly). A white cell analysis and Paul–Bunnell test are indicated. The Paul–Bunnell test, however, may take up to 10 days to become positive.

A white membrane covering one or both tonsils is characteristic and helpful in diagnosis. Hypersensitivity to ampicillin is increased in infectious mononucleosis, and the antibiotic should be avoided as a severe urticaria follows its use. The positive Paul-Bunnell blood test is diagnostic of infections mononucleosis, and atypical mononuclear white cells are increased on the blood film.

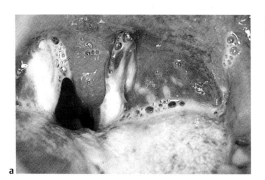

a

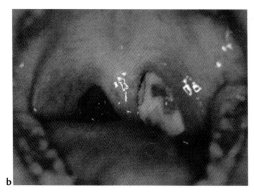

b

Fig. 4.**57a, b Infectious mononucleosis.**

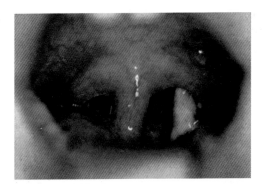

Fig. 4.**58 Infectious mononucleosis in a patient without tonsils.** In this case, the membrane characteristic of infectious mononucleosis is seen either on the lingual tonsil or, as in this case, on a prominent posterior pharyngeal band of lymphoid tissue. A similar white membrane also covers the lymphoid tissue in the postnasal space.

The appearance on examination of the postnasal space may lead to a suspicion of neoplasm. The increase in bulk of the adenoids also causes a "nasal voice," which is sometimes characteristic of infectious mononucleosis.

Oral Candidiasis (Thrush)

Monilia, or oral candidiasis (thrush), is one of the fungal infections of the pharynx. Extensive white areas cover the entire oropharynx, and are not confined to the tonsil. They are either continuous (Fig. 4.**59a**) or punctate (Fig. 4.**59b**). A swab shows *Candida albicans* and confirms the diagnosis. The condition responds to antifungal mouth washes or lozenges containing nystatin or amphotericin. It is commoner in neonates, and may complicate treatment with broad spectrum antibiotics.

Oral candidiasis is one of the commonest upper respiratory tract ***manifestations of AIDS***; unexplained oral fungal infection should make the possibility of AIDS a diagnostic consideration (Fig. 4.**60**). Nasal vestibulitis and cervical lymphadenopathy may be associated findings.

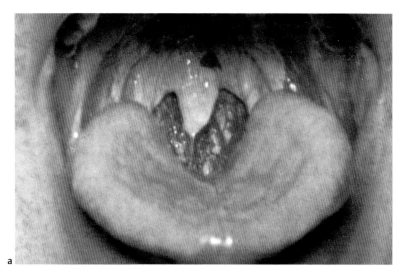

a

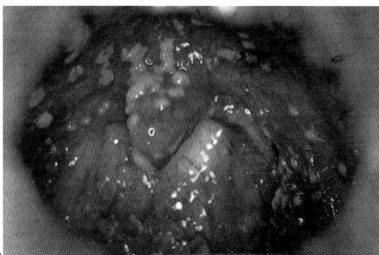

b

Fig. 4.**59a, b Oral candidiasis. a** Extensive continuous white areas covering the oropharynx.
b Extensive punctate white areas covering the oropharynx.

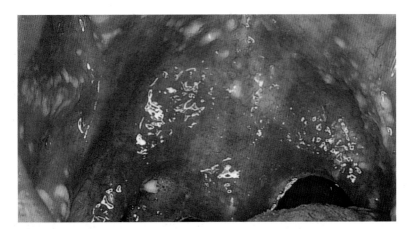

Fig. 4.**60 AIDS-related oral candidiasis.** This is a common presentation of HIV infection. Oral candida is treated with topical or systemic antifungal agents, e. g., nystatin, ketoconazole, or fluconazole. If there is dysphagia with oral candida, esophageal involvement should be suspected.

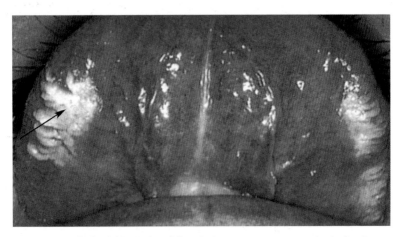

Fig. 4.**61 Hairy leukoplakia.** Oral candidiasis is the commonest presentation in the pharynx of AIDS, but hairy leukoplakia (arrow) is a further presentation on the under surface of this tongue, along with cervical lymphadenopathy.

Oral hairy leukoplakia differs from oral candida in that it is distributed along the lateral borders of the tongue and cannot be scraped off. It is due to Epstein–Barr virus reactivation. Mouth ulcers also occur with HIV infection and good oral hygiene and dental care are important adjuncts to treatment.

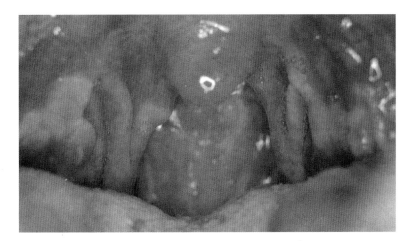

Fig.4.**62 Ulcers on the tonsil and soft palate.** Candida was cultured, but these are ***snail-track ulcers of secondary syphilis.***

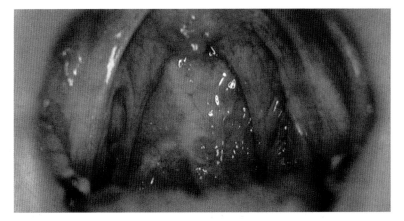

Fig.4.**63 Chronic pharyngitis.** In this condition there is a generalized hyperemia of the pharyngeal mucous membrane, with hyperemic masses of lymphoid tissue on the posterior wall of the oropharynx. A persistent, slightly sore throat is the main symptom. The cause is usually "irritative" rather than due to chronic infection. Environment, occupation, diet, and tobacco are the common factors.

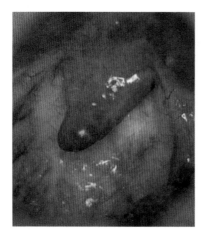

Fig. 4.64 Scleroma with scarring of the soft palate and oropharynx. This is a specific chronic inflammatory disease of the upper respiratory tract mucosa predominantly occurring in Eastern Europe, Asia, and South America. A protracted painless inflammation of the nose (*rhinoscleroma*), pharynx, or larynx is followed after many years by extensive scarring, which is particularly apparent in the oropharynx. Unlike gummatous ulceration, which is a differential diagnosis, scleroma is not destructive, the uvula is preserved, although it may be retracted by scarring into the nasopharynx, and is seen with the postnasal mirror. The histology of the mucosa in scleroma is characteristic and diagnostic.

Tonsillectomy

Tonsillectomy is one of the most frequently performed operations in the world. Stricter indications for operating, however, are reducing the number of tonsillectomies. Recurrent episodes of acute tonsillitis, interfering with school or work, are the main indications. A quinsy or chronic tonsillitis are other indications, along with marked enlargement interfering with the airway.

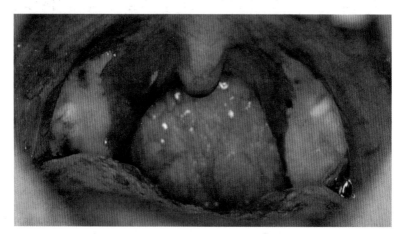

Fig. 4.65 The tonsillar fossae following tonsillectomy. These are covered with a white/yellow membrane for about 10 days until the fossae are epithelialized.

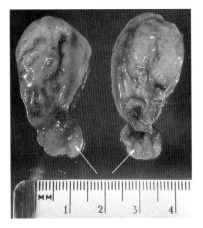

Fig. 4.**66 Tonsils after removal to demonstrate the lingual pole** (arrows). The pole must be included at tonsillectomy. A tonsil remnant may be left inadvertently at this site, giving rise to further infection, but tonsils do not "regrow." Adenoid tissue is, however, not possible to enucleate and remove in toto; it may recur, particularly when removed before age 4.

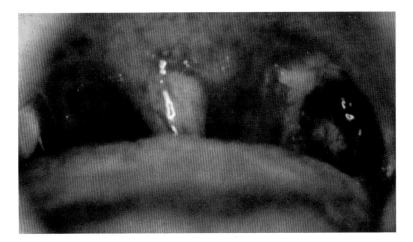

Fig. 4.**67 Secondary infection.** A blood clot in the tonsillar fossa is an important postoperative finding, and almost certainly indicates secondary infection. This occurs between day three and 10, and is associated with bleeding and increased pain. The bleeding is usually scanty and settles when antibiotics control the secondary infection. Severe delayed bleeding after tonsillectomy may occur, however. The finding of a blood clot in a tonsillar fossa must not be ignored.

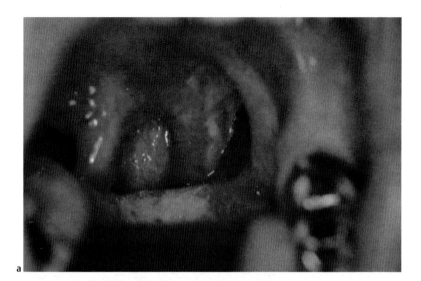

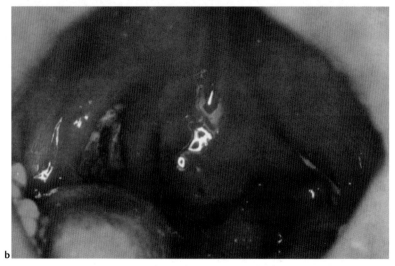

Fig. 4.**68a, b Secondary tonsillar infection with bleeding and bruising of the soft palate.**
This appearance may be related to an excessively traumatic tonsillectomy. An infected blood
clot is present in the tonsillar fossa; removal may cause more bleeding. A tonsillar blood clot
present with primary bleeding, however, should be removed if possible, as this may settle
the bleeding.

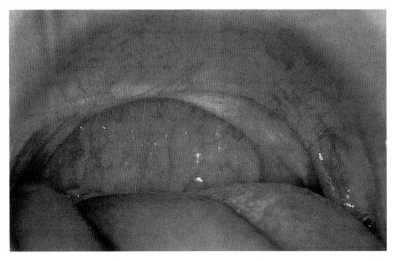

Fig. 4.**69 Guillotine tonsillectomy.** Tonsillectomy today is by dissection with minimal injury to the fauces and surrounding structures. Adept use of the guillotine may also be a rapid and effective surgical technique, but removal of the uvula and fauces is possible in inexperienced hands. Fortunately, postoperative scarring of the palate and uvula is frequently symptom-free. This appearance of the soft palate with conspicuous shortening is similar to that following the uvulopalatoplasty operation for severe snoring (see Fig. 4.**40a, b**).

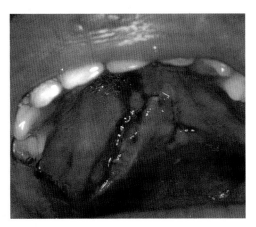

Fig. 4.**70   Palatal trauma.** Laceration to the hard and soft palate are not uncommon. The oft-given advice to children not to "run with a pencil or similar object in their mouth" is intended to offset palatal laceration resulting from a fall. Suturing, however, is usually unnecessary, and unless there is gross mucosal separation, the palate and tongue heal well spontaneously following trauma.

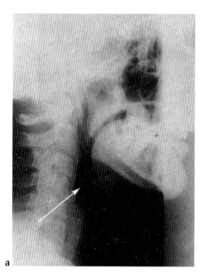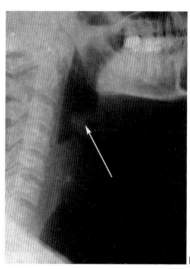

a   b

Fig. 4.**71a, b Epiglottitis.** This is a serious, life-threatening condition and a diagnosis that may be missed. The complaint of a sore throat in an ill patient with a history of dysphagia and fever, often strongly suggestive of a quinsy, *is associated with little amiss on oral examination.* Such a situation strongly suggests epiglottitis, and a lateral soft-tissue radiograph is frequently diagnostic. This is a diagnosis not to be missed, and awareness that it also occurs in children is important. Widespread vaccination against influenza B infection has made epiglottitis in children less common.

The normal narrow contour of the epiglottis (**a**, arrow) is seen to be replaced by a round swelling (**b**, arrow). This condition, if ignored, may lead to stridor, respiratory obstruction, and death if the airway is occluded.

Early diagnosis, hospital admission, and intravenous antibiotic therapy (e. g., cefuroxime) is curative. Close nursing observation of the airway is necessary.

The Larynx

Inflammation of the Larynx

Whether acute or chronic, laryngitis presents with hoarseness and generalized hyperemia of the laryngeal mucous membrane. ***Acute laryngitis*** commonly follows an upper respiratory tract infection, or is traumatic following vocal abuse. Voice rest is the most effective treatment.

Chronic laryngitis may be associated with infection in the upper or lower respiratory tract, but is commonly "irritative" due to occupation and environment, vocal abuse, or tobacco. The unusual laryngitis of ***myxoedema*** must not be forgotten.

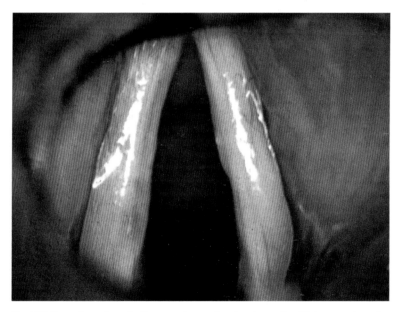

Fig. 4.**72 Normal vocal cords.** These are ivory-colored and smooth with few vessels on the surface. This is the view obtained through a laryngoscope at direct microlaryngoscopy.

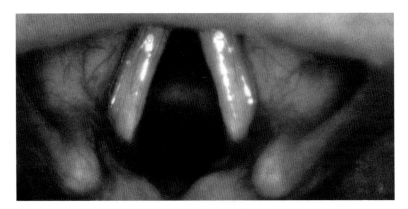

Fig. 4.**73 A fiberoptic endoscopic view of a normal larynx** (see Fig. 1.**61**).

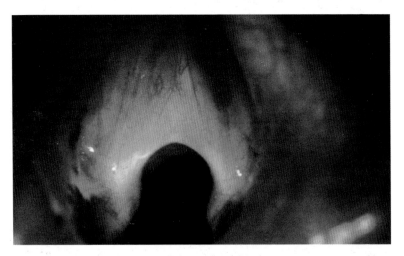

Fig. 4.**74 A laryngeal web.** Congenital abnormalities of the larynx are uncommon. Webbing of varying degrees of severity is one of the commoner developmental abnormalities, and presents as hoarseness. Similar webbing may follow inadvertent trauma at endoscopic surgery to both vocal cords near the anterior commissure. A mucosal web is treated with surgical division. Most webs, however, are deep and fibrous and need an indwelling "keel" after division to avoid recurrence.

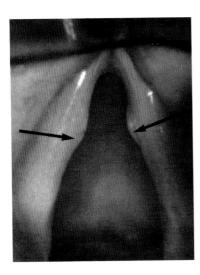

Fig. 4.75 Laryngeal nodules (arrows). A specific and localized type of chronic laryngitis, often seen in professional voice users, is laryngeal nodules (**singer's nodules**). Initially an edema is seen on the vocal cord between the anterior one-third and posterior two-thirds of the cord. Removal of the nodules may be necessary, but attention to the underlying voice production by a speech therapist is the most important aspect of treatment. These nodules are not an uncommon cause of hoarseness in children, particularly of large families involved in competitive shouting (**"screamers" nodules'**). Vocal cord nodules are also seen in those who overuse or misuse their voices.

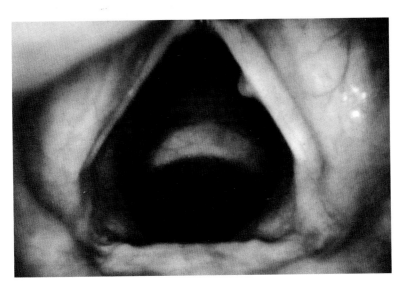

Fig. 4.76 Vocal cord nodule seen through a fiberoptic endoscope. A solitary vocal cord nodule at the characteristic site is not uncommon, although they are usually bilateral and fairly symmetrical.

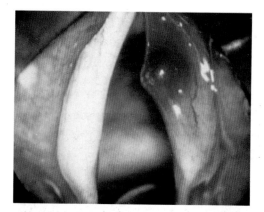

Fig. 4.**77** **Vocal cord nodule with hematoma.** A vocal cord nodule with hematoma formation following vocal abuse.

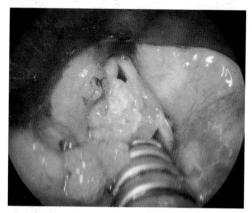

Fig. 4.**78** **Juvenile laryngeal papilloma.**

Recurrent respiratory papillomatosis must be excluded in a hoarse infant or child, for if the hoarseness is ignored, stridor will develop as papillomas accumulate in the laryngeal airway. Nevertheless, vocal cord nodules ("screamers' nodes") are the commonest cause of hoarseness in children.

In juvenile papillomas, multiple wart-like excrescences develop, usually before the age of five, mostly on or around the vocal cords. Recurrence follows removal, but fortunately eventual spontaneous regression is usual. The cause is now established as the human papilloma virus (types 6 and 11), which produces the disease in children who have an HLA-linked T-cell deficit.

Management consists of regular microlaryngoscopy with removal of papillomas using the CO_2 laser or laryngeal microdebrider. The aim is not to achieve radical removal of all the papillomas, but just to maintain a safe airway and as good a voice as possible while awaiting spontaneous resolution, avoiding damage to the underlying laryngeal tissues which might produce scarring and stenosis. In severe cases a tracheostomy may be necessary, but should be avoided if at all possible as papillomas tend to develop around the tracheal stoma and "seed" further down the tracheobronchial tree. In very severe cases adjuvant chemotherapy with interferon may be used.

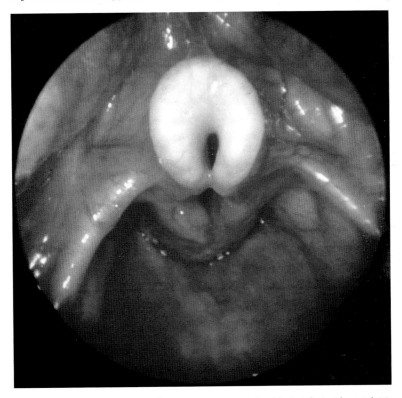

Fig. 4.**79 Laryngomalacia.** This is the commonest cause of stridor in infants. The epiglottis is curled ("omega-shaped") and tightly tethered to the aryepiglottic folds, which are tall and floppy, resulting in supraglottic collapse on inspiration.

Diagnosis can usually be established from the history and confirmed by awake flexible fiberoptic laryngoscopy.

Most cases are mild, no treatment is necessary, and the stridor gradually fades, resolving completely by about age 2. However, 10% of cases are severe with failure to thrive (and often associated gastroesophageal reflux). In these patients an endoscopic aryepiglottoplasty may be required to release the epiglottis and reduce the aryepiglottic folds.

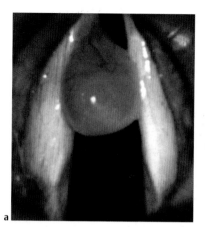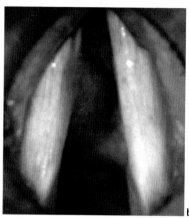

a   b

Fig. 4.**80a, b Pedunculated vocal cord polyp.** A large pedunculated polyp may form on the vocal cord and be missed on examination for it moves above and below the cord on expiration and inspiration. A large polyp (**a**) is less apparent (**b**) when it is below the cord on inspiration.

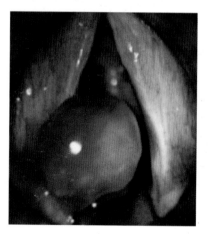

Fig. 4.**81 Intubation granulomas of the larynx.** These result from trauma by the anesthetic tube to the mucosa overlying the vocal process of the arytenoid; they are, therefore, posterior. With the skill that anesthetists have achieved for endotracheal intubation, trauma to this region is uncommon. Granulomas at this site also develop after prolonged vocal abuse has caused a chronic laryngitis in which the epithelium over the vocal process becomes ulcerated ("contact ulcers"). Removal at the pedicle is necessary.

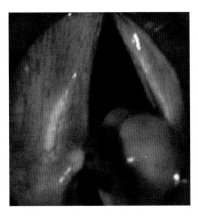

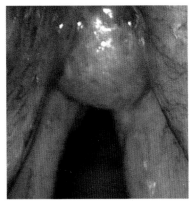

Fig. 4.**82 Granulomas of the larynx excision.** Here the pedicle of the intubation granuloma is being held with forceps. Recurrence frequently follows excision, but laser beam techniques appear to lessen the likelihood. Relatively large lesions can occupy the posterior half of the larynx with minimal voice change. Anteriorly in the larynx, however, small lesions cause conspicuous voice change.

Fig. 4.**83 Polyp at the anterior commissure.** This site is not always easy to see on indirect laryngoscopy for it may be partly obscured by the tubercle of the epiglottis. The laryngoscope is placed against the tubercle, displacing it forwards and a clear view is obtained.

A small lesion near or at the anterior commissure of the larynx may produce conspicuous hoarseness. However, a larger lesion posteriorly in the larynx may not produce such a conspicuous voice change.

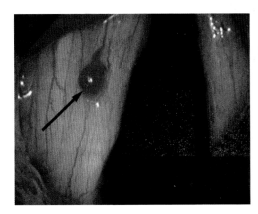

Fig. 4.**84 Hemangiomas** (arrow). These are uncommon vocal cord lesions and if small may cause no hoarseness or bleeding, and be a chance finding on examination. Laser surgery promises to be the effective treatment for larger hemangiomas.

These hemangiomas may be associated with similar lesions in the head and neck in children (Fig. 3.**4a,b**).

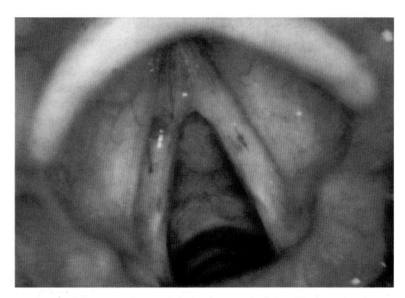

Fig. 4.**85 Acute laryngitis** showing slight hyperemia and edema of both vocal cords seen with the fiberoptic endoscope.

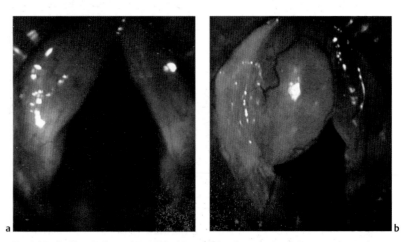

Fig. 4.**86a, b Chronic laryngitis.** With this condition, hyperemia of the mucous membrane may be associated with other changes in the larynx. Edema of the margin of the vocal cords is common (Reinke's edema), so that the free margin is polypoid and a large sessile polyp may form. The edema, although affecting both cords, may be more marked on one side (**b**).

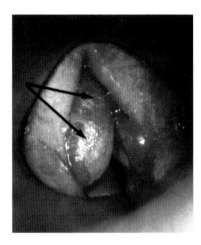

Fig. 4.**87 Hypertrophy of the ventricular bands.** Hypertrophy of the ventricular bands is another finding in chronic laryngitis and they may meet in the mid-line on phonation, producing a characteristic hoarseness. **Reinke's edema** is also present (arrows). Microlaryngoscopy and surgical excision of the edematous margins is effective with dissection or the laser beam. Excision to the anterior commissure is made on one cord only to avoid webbing.

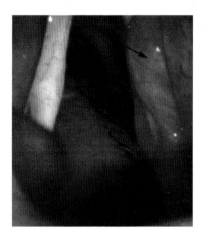

Fig. 4.**88 Prolapse of the ventricular mucous membrane** (arrow). This may also occur in chronic laryngitis and presents as a supraglottic swelling. A supraglottic cyst or carcinoma must be excluded.

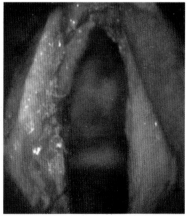

Fig. 4.**89 Long-standing chronic laryngitis.** The mucous membrane may become extremely hypertrophic with white patches (leukoplakia). Histologically, the white patches represent areas of keratosis which may precede malignant change and be reported as carcinoma in situ. This patient had smoked over 60 cigarettes a day for 50 years.

Neoplasms of the Larynx

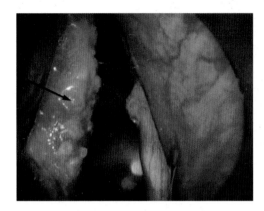

Fig. 4.**90 Carcinoma of the vocal cord.** This usually occurs in smokers. The indurated leukoplakia on this vocal cord (arrow) is a well-differentiated squamous cell carcinoma that has arisen as a result of chronic laryngitis with hyperkeratosis.

The prognosis for vocal cord carcinoma with radiotherapy is excellent, with a cure rate of over 90 % for early lesions. The voice returns to normal, as does the appearance of the vocal cord.

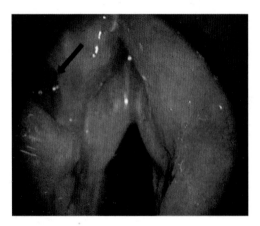

Fig. 4.**91 Supraglottic squamous cell carcinoma.** Carcinoma of the larynx commonly involves the vocal cord (glottic carcinoma), but lesions may develop below the cord (subglottic) or above the cord (supraglottic). The ulcerated area of granulation tissue above the edematous vocal cord in this case is a squamous cell carcinoma (arrow).

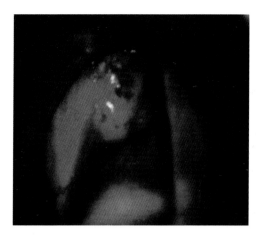

Fig.4.**92** **Subglottic squamous cell carcinoma.** The prognosis for supraglottic and subglottic carcinoma is worse than for glottic carcinoma, for hoarseness is delayed until the cord is involved and the greater vascularity and lymphatic drainage above and below the cord predisposes to earlier metastasis.

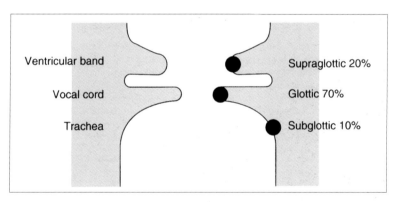

Ventricular band

Vocal cord

Trachea

Supraglottic 20%

Glottic 70%

Subglottic 10%

Fig.4.**93 Carcinoma of the larynx.** 70% of laryngeal carcinomas affect the vocal cords.

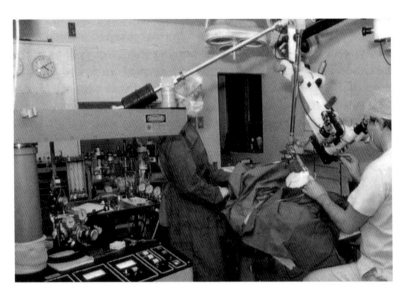

Fig. 4.**94** The laser beam for surgical excision. This may prove to be the technique of choice for certain lesions in the upper respiratory tract. In this case it is being used at microlaryngoscopy to excise an intubation granuloma (see Fig. 4.**81**). The laser is now widely used for the removal of tongue (see Fig. 4.**32**) and pharyngeal lesions, particularly hemangiomas and other vascular lesions. The laser also appears to have advantages for excision of juvenile papillomas, intubation granulomas, and possible laryngeal webs. Use of the operating microscope ensures precise excision with the cold steel microdebrider or with the laser beam, and causes less tissue damage than cautery or diathermy.

Laryngeal Surgery

Laryngectomy

Nearly all cases of early carcinoma of the vocal cord are cured with radiotherapy or laser surgery. Disease, however, may remain with extensive cord carcinomas, with supraglottic or subglottic lesions, or with carcinoma of the pyriform fossa or epiglottis.

Partial laryngectomy (laryngofissure, extended laryngofissure, or supraglottic laryngectomy) gives adequate resection of some laryngeal carcinomas, but frequently a **total laryngectomy** is required. This radical surgery, which may be associated with a **neck dissection** if the nodes are involved, means a permanent tracheostome, and an alternative method of speech has to be developed. Fistula speech, using a valve placed between the trachea and neopharynx at laryngectomy, is the most frequently employed surgical speech technique.

Conservative laryngectomy (supraglottic or hemilaryngectomy) aims in the smaller laryngeal cancers to preserve part or all of the vocal cords and to avoid a tracheostome, so that laryngeal voice is preserved. For those who are unable to speak after total laryngectomy, or as a primary procedure with laryngectomy, a valve fitted between the tracheosteome and esophagus enables air to be redirected with a more normal voice production (Blom–Singer valve).

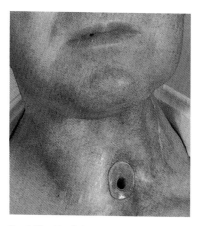

Fig. 4.**95** **Total laryngectomy with left radical neck dissection.**

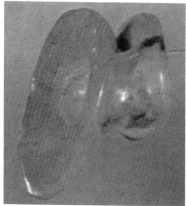

Fig. 4.**96** **Stomal stud.** Stenosis of the tracheosteome is sometimes a postoperative problem, and a small stomal stud can be used.

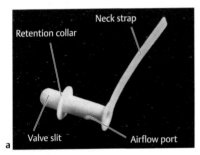
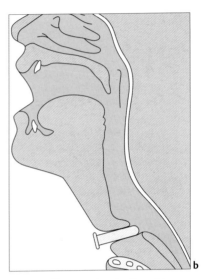

Fig. 4.**97a, b a The Blom–Singer voice prosthesis** is usually inserted at the time of laryng-ectomy. **b** The prosthesis shown diagrammatically and positioned into the new opening to the esophagus at the top of the tracheosteome.

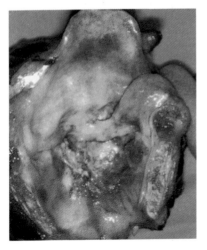

Fig. 4.**98 Laryngectomy specimen.** This shows a large laryngeal carcinoma extend-ing above and below the right vocal cord and across to the left side of the larynx. It also shows the hyoid, thyroid, and cricoid cartilages and upper rings of trachea, which are removed at laryngectomy.

Hoarseness

Hoarseness may be due to ***paralysis of one vocal cord***, the left being more commonly involved. Lack of cord movement on phonation is diagnosed on indirect laryngoscopy or fiberoptic laryngoscopy. Although temporary idiopathic cord palsy is the single most common cause, involvement of the left recurrent laryngeal nerve in chest disease must be excluded. Any hilar lymph node lesion in the region of the aortic arch may involve this nerve, such as secondaries from lung carcinoma. The enlarged left atrium of mitral stenosis may also press on the left recurrent laryngeal nerve and cause hoarseness, as may an aortic aneurysm or the enlarged pulmonary artery of pulmonary hypertension.

The recurrent laryngeal nerves are also occasionally damaged in the neck by severe external injury, or by thyroid carcinoma or surgery. Central lesions, or lesions near the jugular foramen involving the vagus, may also cause cord paralysis, and hoarseness is one of the symptoms of posterior inferior cerebellar artery thrombosis.

A neck MRI scan is a necessary investigation to exclude a thyroid neoplasm, which may involve the recurrent laryngeal nerve. If the scan shows a thyroid gland mass or adjacent lymph node, a fine needle aspiration (see p. 264) is required.

Hoarseness, particularly a whispered voice with normal larynx, is a functional voice problem. ***Nonorganic aphonia*** is not uncommon in young women, and stems from a superficial psychiatric upset. Treatment from the speech therapist is usually effective without referral to a psychiatrist being necessary. Curious alterations in the voice or hoarseness may also be due to a nonorganic dysphonia.

Phonosurgery

Microsurgical techniques are effective to restore normal quality of a hoarse voice. Minute lesions on or within the vocal cord can be excised or enucleated with precision.

Phonosurgery is of particular use for established vocal cord palsy. The voice is weak and "breathy" because the glottis does not fully "close" on phonation. Techniques to medialize or increase the bulk of the immobile cord enable full closure of the glottis and normal or near-normal voice to be achieved.

Stroboscopy

Stroboscopy is a further technique for demonstrating laryngeal pathology with the endoscope and video camera (see Fig. 4.**99a, b**). The rapid movements of the vocal cords during phonation can be seen magnified and in slow motion. Minimal cord lesions causing voice change which were hitherto undetectable can be diagnosed and treated, for example, small nodes and cysts within the vocal cord.

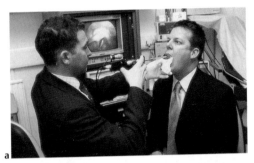

a

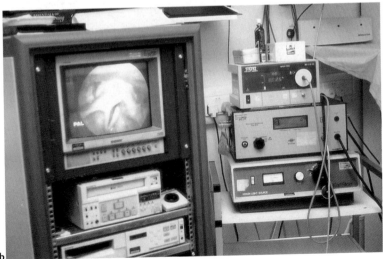

b

Fig. 4.**99a, b Stroboscopy** is a further technique for demonstrating laryngeal pathology with the endoscope and video camera.

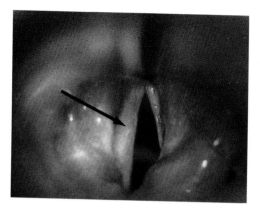

Fig. 4.**100** **Left vocal cord palsy.** The paralyzed vocal cord is seen to lie near the mid-line (arrow) and undergoes no movement on phonation at indirect laryngoscopy (see Fig. 1.**60**). The paralyzed vocal cord is seen to fall medially towards the mid-line and inferiorly, so it is below (inferior to) the cord with normal movement.

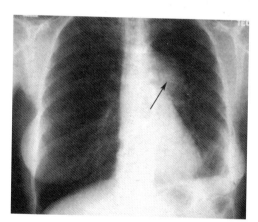

Fig. 4.**101** **Radiograph of aortic aneurysm** (arrow). Pressure on the left recurrent laryngeal nerve causes nerve palsy and hoarseness.

An enlarged hilar lymph node secondary to a lung carcinoma in this site is a common cause of hoarseness due to left vocal cord palsy.

Microsurgery of the Larynx

The use of the microscope for direct laryngoscopy has greatly increased the scope and precision of laryngeal surgery. All small benign lesions of the larynx are excised with this technique. Biopsies of malignant disease can be taken accurately from the suspicious area with minimal damage to adjacent tissue.

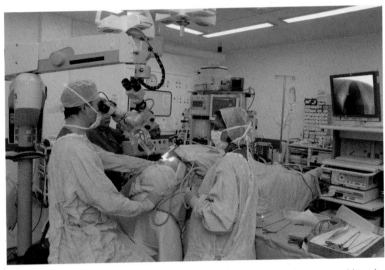

Fig. 4.**102 Microlaryngoscopy.** The holder for the laryngoscope is clamped, enabling the surgeon to have both hands free for instrumentation. Images can be recorded digitally and shown on the monitor for teaching purposes. Cold light instruments give bright, reliable illumination, and the development of a light-transmitting glass fiber cable has been another advance in endoscopy.

Tracheostomy

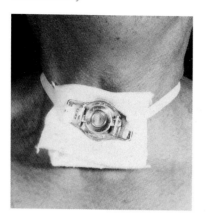

Fig. 4.**103 A patient after tracheostomy** (with speaking valve).

Obstruction of the larynx causes stridor, and may necessitate a tracheostomy. Acute inflammatory conditions of the upper respiratory tract (e.g., epiglottis), foreign bodies or neoplasms limiting the airway are the commonest causes of stridor.

Tracheostomy is also required for respiratory failure due to central depression of the respiratory center, for example, strokes, barbiturate poisoning, head injury, poliomyelitis, or tetanus. Multiple rib fractures or severe chest infections may require tracheostomy. Tracheostomy enables breathing to be controlled by an intermittent positive pressure respirator, and bronchial secretions can be removed with suction. A prolonged obstruction of the glottis may occur with juvenile papillomas, severe trauma to the larynx, or bilateral cord palsies, making a permanent tracheostomy necessary. *A tracheostomy tube with a speaking valve* allows air to enter during inspiration, but closes on expiration so that air passes through the larynx for phonation.

Emergency tracheostomy may be a difficult operation, particularly if done under local anesthetic when a general anesthetic with intubation is not practical. An opening into the trachea through the cricothyroid membrane offers a simpler and more direct relief for upper respiratory tract obstruction.

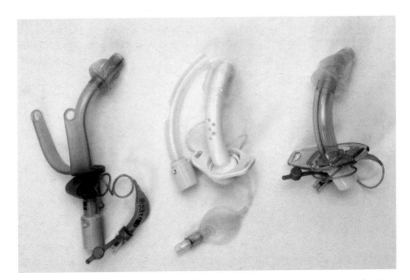

Fig. 4.**104 Plastic tracheostomy tubes.** Right: the standard cuffed tracheostomy tube. Center: this tube has a coaxial flange with an inner tube fenestration to allow speech. Left: an adjustable flanged cuffed tube.

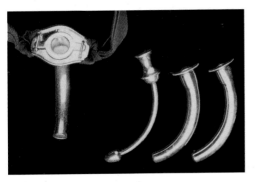

Fig. 4.**105   Silver tracheostomy tubes in common use** (Negus).

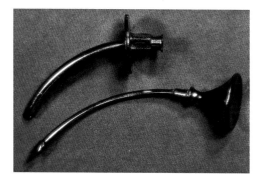

Fig.4.**106** **Cricothyrotomy cannula with trocar.** This instrument has been devised for emergency operations. A tracheostomy can be performed later when the emergency of the acute obstruction is past.

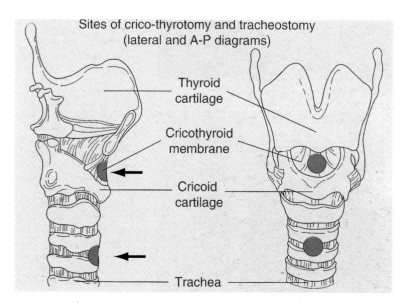

Sites of crico-thyrotomy and tracheostomy
(lateral and A-P diagrams)

Thyroid
cartilage

Cricothyroid
membrane

Cricoid
cartilage

Trachea

Fig.4.**107 Tracheostomy.** Openings are usually made between the 2nd and 3rd tracheal rings. A "higher" tracheostomy predisposes to stenosis of the larynx in the subglottic region. The airway is most accessible and superficial at the level of the cricothyroid membrane, and in acute laryngeal obstruction an opening through the membrane will restore the airway. The cricothyrotomy opening is, however, for an emergency, and is only temporary. Indwelling tubes at this site lead to subglottic stenosis of the larynx.

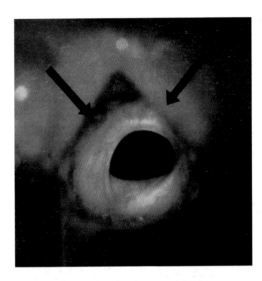

Fig. 4.108 Subglottic stenoses. Slightly hyperemic cords (arrows) with an area of ring-like stenosis below the vocal cords can be seen in this patient. This stenosis followed trauma, partly related to a road traffic accident in which the trachea was injured, and also related to a high tracheostomy through the first tracheal ring. Dilation is rarely effective for this type of cicatricial stenosis, and excision of the stenotic area of the trachea with end-to-end anastomosis or grafting procedures are necessary. Subglottic stenosis is also a complication of prolonged endotracheal intubation.

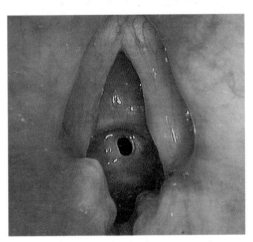

Fig. 4.109 Subglottic stenosis in babies and children. This may be congenital due to a grossly thickened cricoid cartilage, or acquired secondary to neonatal intubation with consequent cicatricial fibrosis.

Dilatation is ineffective, and endoscopic laser treatment is appropriate for only the mildest cases.

Most of these children will require a tracheostomy, followed by a laryngotracheal reconstruction with costal cartilage grafting.

The Hypopharynx and Esophagus

Globus Pharyngeus

This is a very common condition in which the patient, not infrequently a young girl, complains of a sensation of a lump in the throat. The site indicated is the cricoid region.

When taking the history, a helpful direct question is to ask whether the lump is most apparent on swallowing food, fluid, or saliva. The patient with globus will consistently reply that saliva is the problem, and that the symptom occurs between meals.

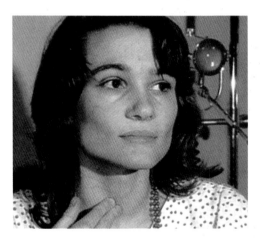

Fig. 4.**110 Globus pharyngeus.** The patient is indicating the region of the cricoid cartilage which is the site of discomfort with globus pharyngeus.

The symptom of discomfort —not pain, in the region of the cricoid is not infrequently associated with nasal symptoms of postnasal discharge or chronic rhinitis where frequent swallowing predisposes and accentuates the globus symptom.

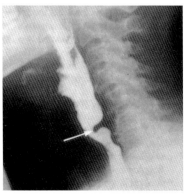

Fig. 4.**111 Barium swallow.** Globus pharyngeus is a psychosomatic condition, but there is a demonstrable spasm of the cricopharyngeus on barium swallow, where the barium column is seen to be "nipped." Overattention by the patient perpetuates the spasm, and usually reassurance and explanation are the only treatments required.

Globus pharyngeus is not necessarily nonorganic, and "globus hystericus" is a misnomer. It is a condition that may call for investigation, particularly in the older age group, when it may be the presenting symptom of disease in the esophagus or stomach. Hiatus hernia and esophageal reflux commonly cause cricopharyngeal spasm, and gastric ulcers and neoplasms may also present with globus. A barium swallow and meal is, therefore, an important investigation (Fig. 4.**111**). Cervical osteoarthritis (Fig. 4.**112a, b**, arrow) with marked changes in the region of the 6th cervical vertebra may also give rise to globus.

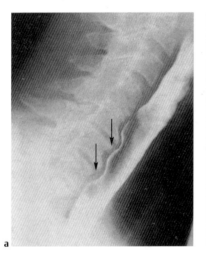
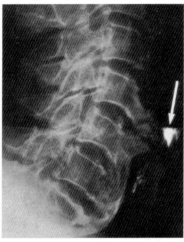

a   b

Fig. 4.**112a, b Cervical osteoarthritis. a** Projection of cervical osteophytes into the postcricoid region of the upper esophagus (arrows) causes cricopharyngeal spasm and the symptom of globus. **b** In this radiograph, gross osteophytes have caused "nipping" of the barium (arrow) by the cricopharyngeus muscle.

Pharyngeal Pouch (see p. 256)

This is a herniation of mucous membrane through the posterior fibers of the inferior constrictor muscle above the cricopharyngeus, usually occurring in old age. The defect predisposing to its development is a failure of coordinated relaxation of the cricopharyngeus on swallowing. A pouch is frequently associated with a hiatus hernia.

A small pouch may cause no symptoms, but when large, dysphagia develops, varying from slight to absolute. There is regurgitation of undigested food, gurgling may be heard in the neck after eating, or a swelling may be seen, laterally in the neck, usually on the left.

The pouch accumulates food, and spillage into the respiratory tract may cause coughing. A pouch may present with respiratory disease—either bronchitis, apical fibrosis simulating tuberculosis, or acute pulmonary infection (bronchitis, bronchopneumonia, or a lung abscess).

The barium swallow is the only investigation required to confirm the diagnosis of pharyngeal pouch. If symptoms are marked, surgery is needed. ***Endoscopic stapling techniques*** with division of the party wall has replaced a neck incision with pouch excision and repair. Rarely, a carcinoma occurs within the lumen of a pharyngeal pouch.

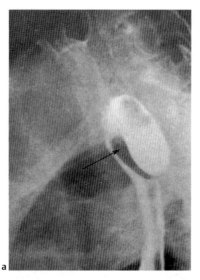

a

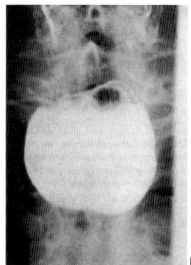

b

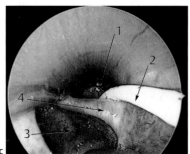

c

Fig. 4.**113a–c Pharyngeal pouch. a, b** Barium swallow. **c** At endoscopy the esophagus (1) with esophageal tube are seen (2). The lumen of the pouch (3) and the party wall (4) which is stabled and incised using an endoscopic staple gun.

Foreign Bodies

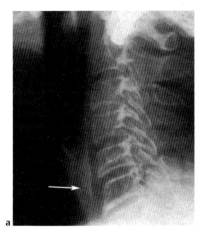

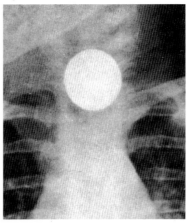

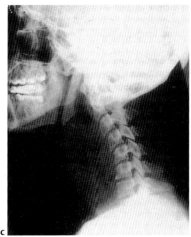

Fig. 4.**114a–c Foreign bodies in the esophagus.** Foreign bodies, such as bones, coins, pins, dentures, and small toys, may impact in the upper third of the esophagus. A history of possible foreign impaction must not be ignored as esophageal perforation leads to cervical cellulitis and mediastinitis, which may be fatal.

Air seen on radiograph behind the pharynx and esophagus is diagnostic of a perforation. Persistent dysphagia, pain referred to the neck or back, pain on inspiration, and fever all suggest a foreign body.

Chest radiography and radiography of the neck are essential investigations, but even if negative, persistent symptoms are suspicious and esophagoscopy is necessary. However, coins which pass the cricopharyngeus usually traverse the rest of the gut, and rarely require removal.

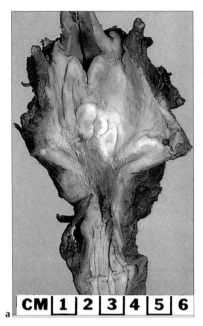

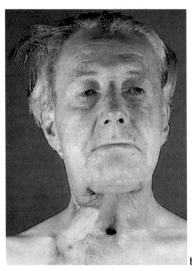

Fig. 4.**115a, b Carcinoma of the pyriform fossa and upper esophagus.** The presenting signs are dysphagia for solids and pain, commonly referred to the ear.

There is early metastasis to the cervical nodes. A carcinoma involving mainly the medial wall of the pyriform fossa causes hoarseness.

The prognosis is not good, particularly with upper esophageal carcinoma, whether treatment is with radiotherapy or surgery. Resection for these carcinomas involves a pharyngolaryngectomy and the replacement or reconstruction of the cervical esophagus poses technical problems. Immediate replacement with stomach or colon, mobilized and brought through the thorax and sutured to the pharynx, is one technique.

The delayed use of neck and chest myocutaneous flaps is an alternative method of reconstruction. Microvascular surgical techniques have enabled immediate reconstruction with a section of the ileum, which is a further option.

5 The Head and Neck

Salivary Glands

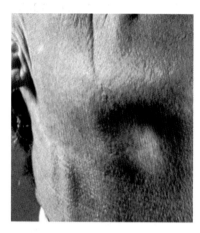

Fig. 5.**1 Submandibular calculus.** A calculus obstructing the submandibular duct causes painful and intermittent enlargement of the gland. The swelling occurs on eating and regresses slowly. Secondary infection in the gland leads to persistent tender swelling of the gland. The swelling in the submandibular triangle is visible and palpable bimanually with one finger in the mouth.

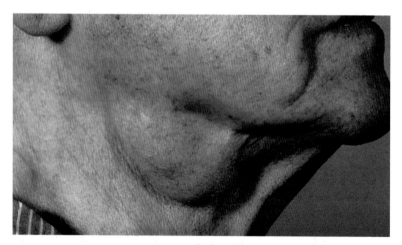

Fig. 5.**2 Grossly enlarged submandibular gland.** This develops if an impacted calculus is ignored. A neoplasm of the submandibular gland is the differential diagnosis if the enlargement is persistent and there is no evidence of a calculus on radiograph. The nodular surface and the firm, nontender character on palpation of this gland are also suggestive of a neoplasm, commonly a ***pleomorphic adenoma*** or adenoid cystic carcinoma.

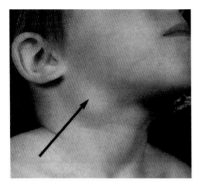

Fig. 5.3 Tonsillary lymph node enlargement. A tonsillar lymph node enlargement (arrow) may be similar to an enlarged submandibular gland. This node is frequently palpable in children, being more conspicuous at times of tonsillar or upper respiratory tract infection, and may become very obvious, as in this case. The node is soft and tender.

Exact location of the site is important: It is *posterior to the submandibular triangle* at the angle of the mandible, and not within the submandibular triangle.

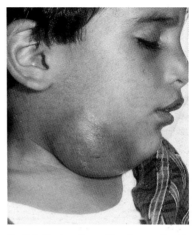

Fig. 5.4 Abscess formation in a submandibular triangle lymph node secondary to dental infection. *Mumps* may also cause a tender submandibular swelling, and an enlarged lymph node in the submandibular triangle, secondary to dental infection, simulates gland involvement.

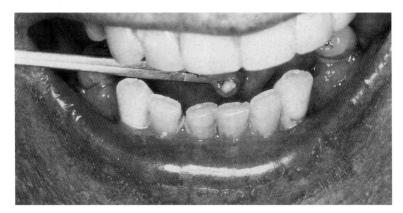

Fig. 5.5 Submandibular calculus impacted at the orifice of the duct. This is easily removed with local anesthesia in the outpatients.

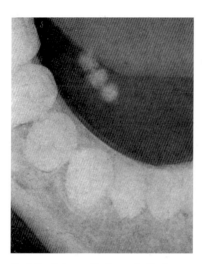

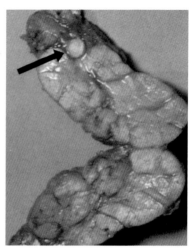

Fig. 5.**6   Submandibular calculi demonstrated on radiograph** impacted in the duct. An anterior calculus may be removed by incision over the duct in the floor of the mouth, a suture being placed posterior to the calculus to prevent "slippage backwards" towards the gland.

Fig. 5.**7 Excision of the submandibular gland** (specimen) is required for calculi impacted in the duct or within the gland (arrow). Care is taken in this operation to preserve the mandibular branch of the facial nerve which crosses the submandibular triangle to supply the muscles of the angle of the mouth.

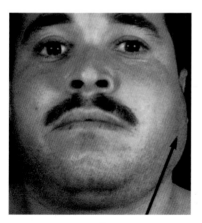

Fig. 5.**8 Mixed parotid tumor (pleomorphic adenoma) (arrow).** These present as a firm, smooth, nontender swelling. The growth is slow, so the history may be long. The bulk of the parotid lies in the neck posterior to the ramus of the mandible, and parotid tumors do not usually cause predominantly facial swelling.

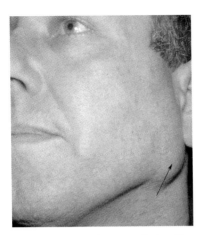

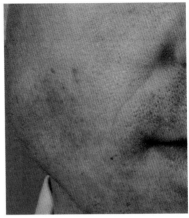

Fig. 5.**9 Parotid swelling.** A softer swelling in the tail of the parotid (arrow) may be an *adenolymphoma* (Warthin's tumor), a benign tumor of salivary gland tissue within a parotid lymph node. The pleomorphic adenoma is a low-grade malignant tumor, and is commonly in the superficial lobe of the parotid. The treatment is a **superficial parotidectomy** with preservation of the facial nerve. A soft parotid swelling with a short history and a partial or complete facial palsy is probably an adenoid cystic carcinoma or higher-grade malignant tumor of the parotid gland, requiring total parotidectomy with sacrifice of the facial nerve and radiotherapy.

Fig. 5.**10 Congenital hypertrophy of the masseter muscle.** Careful palpation follows observation of a swelling, and what appears as a parotid mass here is palpable as a congenital hypertrophy of the masseter muscle.

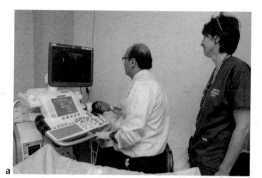

Fig. 5.**11a, b Ultrasound-guided fine needle aspiration (US-FNA)** cytology is a frequently used investigation for neck swellings. Findings on color flow Doppler also help diagnose neck swellings, and when combined with FNA may avoid the necessity of an open biopsy.

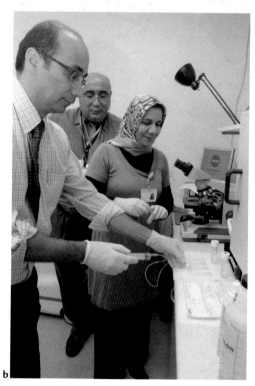

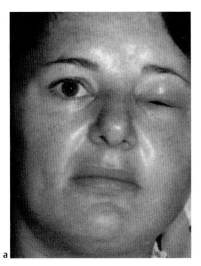
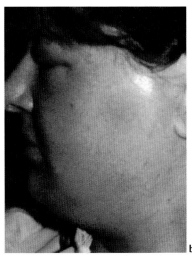

a
b

Fig. 5.**12a, b Mumps.** Acute viral parotitis is a common infection, and the diagnosis is usually obvious. Well-defined tender swelling of the parotid gland, first on one side and shortly after on the other, with associated trismus and malaise, are characteristic. However, mumps can be deceptive when it remains unilateral and the swelling is not strictly confined to the parotid. In this case of mumps (**a, b**), the swelling involved the side of the face, causing lid and facial edema. Unilateral total deafness is a complication of mumps.

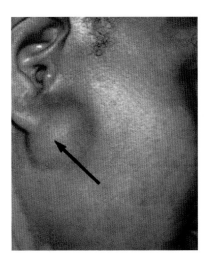

Fig. 5.**13 Sebaceous cyst.** A swelling in the parotid region (arrow), but on the face suggests another diagnosis. There is a small punctum on the swelling in this picture, diagnostic of a sebaceous cyst.

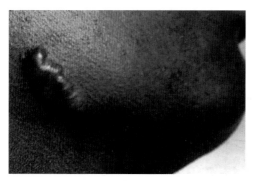

Fig. 5.**14 Sebaceous cyst on the face.** Minor lesions such as sebaceous cysts present a problem on the face when excision is needed. Particular care is needed to enucleate these cysts meticulously, through incisions made within the relaxed skin tension lines. It may also be necessary to "break-up" the straight incision line so that it is less obvious. A **keloid** is a further concern. This followed excision of a sebaceous cyst in the upper neck.

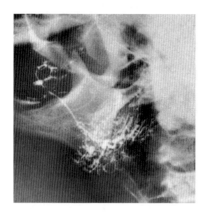

Fig. 5.**15 Sialectasis of the parotid gland.** This presents as intermittent episodes of painful swelling. Calculi in the parotid duct are uncommon, and are not easily demonstrated on radiograph. An intraoral view is necessary.

A sialogram confirms sialectasis, and the punctate dilations of the parotid ducts are similar in appearance to bronchiectasis. The parotid swelling with sialectasis is often infrequent and mild, and triggered by certain foods.

There is no simple treatment; superficial parotidectomy is reserved for the rare, severe cases.

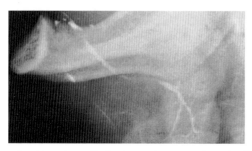

Fig. 5.**16 Normal submandibular sialogram.** The pattern of ducts not involved with sialectasis is demonstrated. A parotid sialogram is not difficult to perform, since the duct orifice opposite the second upper molar tooth is obvious and can be made more apparent by massaging over the parotid gland to cause a visible flow of saliva. The submandibular duct orifice anteriorly in the floor of the mouth is not obvious; cannulation for sialography may be difficult.

Swelling of the Neck

Congenital Neck Swellings

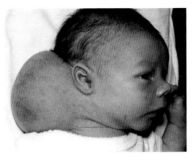

Fig. 5.**17 Lymphangiomas** are developmental anomalies in which the lymphatic and venous channels fail to connect, resulting in fluid-filled spaces which expand. Lesions may be macrocystic with large compressible elements (previously called cystic hygroma); microscopic cysts are smaller and firmer. These lesions are often seen at birth and may be very large, causing airway obstruction. They may, however, present later in childhood, enlarging rapidly with upper respiratory tract infections.

Lymphangiomas do not involute spontaneously. However, small lesions may simply be observed. Sclerotherapy and surgery are other options. Care must be taken to avoid damaging the neurovascular structures as these are benign and tend to recur.

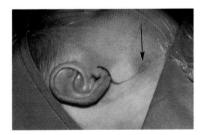

Fig. 5.**18 First arch anomaly.** This rare branchial cleft anomaly presents as an opening on the line between the tragus and the hyoid bone (arrow). The upper end of the fistula is in the region of the external ear canal. The fistulae are skin lined and commonly become infected and discharged. Surgical excision is necessary via a parotidectomy-type incision to include the lower fistulous opening. Care must be taken in excising the fistula to avoid injury to the facial nerve, which may lie close to the fistula's tract.

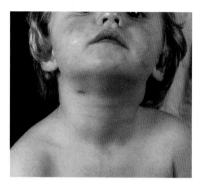

Fig. 5.**19a Second branchial fistula**, the most common of the branchial arch anomalies. The lower opening lies anterior to the sternomastoid muscle. The tract passes between the internal and external carotid arteries and communicates with the pharynx often through the tonsil. The fistula discharges fluid and often becomes infected. Surgery to remove the complete tract is frequently necessary.

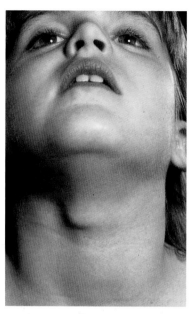

Fig. 5.**19b Thyroglossal duct cysts** are the most common congenital neck cysts. This midline cyst and tract are formed in the path of thyroid migration in embryogenesis and are always related to the hyoid. Failure to remove the central part of the hyoid will result in recurrence.

Inflammatory Neck Swellings

The spread of dental infection must be remembered as a possible cause of inflammatory neck swelling.

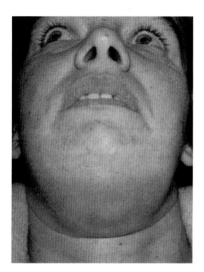

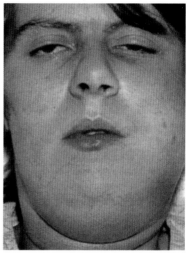

Fig. 5.**20 Ludwig's angina.** An indurated, tender, mid-line inflammation is characteristic of Ludwig's angina. Bimanual palpation reveals a characteristic woody firmness of the normally soft tissues of the floor of the mouth, which is an early sign. This acute infection may spread from the apices of the lower incisors, in this case following extraction.

In the preantibiotic era this condition was serious, because spread of infection involved the larynx and caused the acute onset of stridor. This complication is still to be remembered, although extensive neck incisions to relieve pus under pressure are rarely necessary, and the response to intramuscular penicillin is good.

Fig. 5.**21 Cervical cellulitis** may develop from a dental abscess in the lower molars and involve the neck laterally.

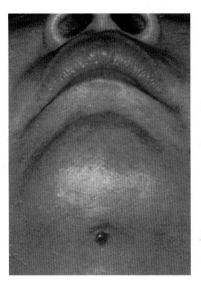

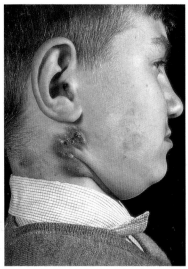

Fig. 5.**22 Submental sinus.** A chronic, localized, mid-line infection under the chin is probably a submental sinus. This recurrent mass of granulation tissue formed at the opening of a sinus, leading to *apical infection in a lower incisor tooth.*

Fig. 5.**23 Tuberculous cervical abscesses.** These are uncommon in countries where cattle are tuberculin tested, as intake of infected milk is the usual cause. A chronic, discharging neck abscess in the posterior triangle is characteristic of tuberculosis. Firm, nontender nodes without sinus formation in the same site are also suggestive of tuberculosis. Chemotherapy alone usually fails to control this condition, and excision of the nodes or chronic abscesses is required.

Mid-line Neck Swellings

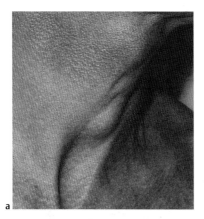

a

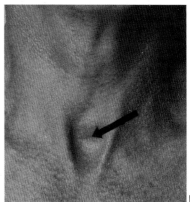

b

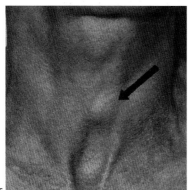

c

Fig. 5.**24 Thyroglossal cyst.** This is a midline neck swelling forming in the remnant of the thyroglossal tract (**a**). The swelling is commonly between the thyroid and hyoid, but suprahyoid cysts also occur. The convexity of the hyoid bone and thyroid cartilage push the cyst to one side, so it may not be strictly mid-line. The cyst moves on swallowing and on protrusion of the tongue (**b, c,** arrows). It is usually nontender but may present with recurrent episodes of acute swelling and tenderness.

Treatment is excision with removal of the body of the hyoid bone and tract (Sistrunk's procedure). Failure to excise the body of the hyoid predisposes to recurrence for the thyroglossal tract extends in a loop deep to the hyoid bone.

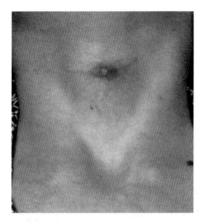

Fig. 5.**25 Thyroglossal cyst.** Excision of the cyst alone, without the tract and body of the hyoid bone, leads to recurrence. The cyst remnant causes inflammation and discharge at the scar. This appearance is characteristic of an inadequately excised thyroglossal cyst.

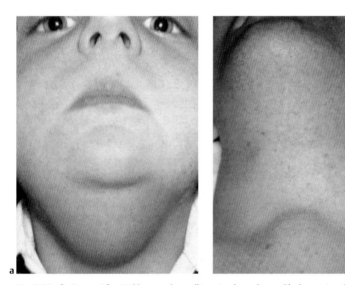

a   b

Fig. 5.**26a, b Dermoids.** Mid-line neck swellings in the submandibular region (**a**) or suprasternal region (**b**) are commonly dermoids.

Lateral Neck Swellings

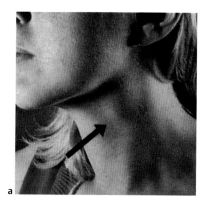

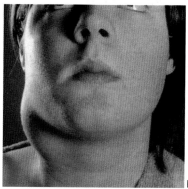

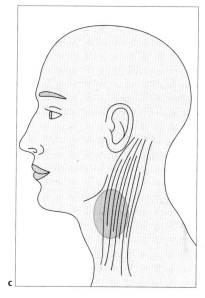

Fig. 5.**27a–c Branchial cyst** (**a**, arrow; **b**). This has a consistent site, is smooth, and, if there is no secondary infection, nontender. It lies between the upper one-third and lower two-thirds of the anterior border of the sternomastoid, and is deep to and partly concealed by this muscle (**c**). It can be large by the time it presents. When excised, the deep surface is found to be closely related to the internal jugular vein.

A metastatic lymph node from the thyroid, upper respiratory tract (e.g., naso-pharynx) or postcricoid region, and swellings of neurogenous origin (chemodecto-mas, neurofibromas, neuroblastomas) are among the important differential diagnoses of a lateral neck swelling. The ubiquitous lip-oma is also not uncommon in the neck, and in children the cystic hygroma is to be re-membered. Hodgkin's disease also fre-quently presents with an enlarged cervical lymph node.

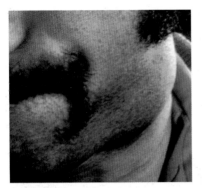

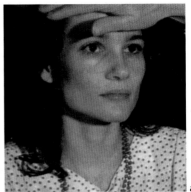

Fig. 5.28 **Laryngocele.** This is an unusual neck swelling that the patient can inflate with the Valsalva maneuver. It is an enlargement of the laryngeal saccule into the neck between hyoid and thyroid cartilage. It tends to occur in musicians who play wind instruments, or in glass blowers. Infection may develop in laryngoceles (a pyolaryngocele), and presents as an acute neck swelling often with hoarseness and stridor.

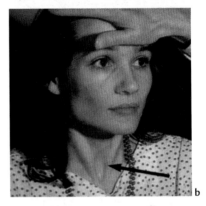

a

b

Fig. 5.**29a–c   Test for accessory cranial ▶ nerve (XI) function.** The sternomastoid muscle is supplied by the accessory nerve. If the patient is asked to press the forehead against the examiner's hand (**a**), the sternal attachments of the muscle stand out (**b**, arrow). When cranial nerve X is inactive, the sternal head on the side of the lesion remains flat (**c**, arrow).

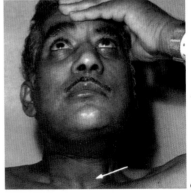

c

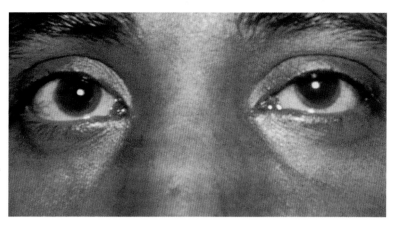

Fig. 5.**30 Horner's syndrome.** Pressure on the sympathetic nerve trunk in the neck, particularly by malignant disease, causes changes in the eye. Ptosis, with a small pupil, is apparent in the patient's left eye; this is also associated with an enophthalmos and a lack of sweating. With a cervical swelling, examination should exclude Horner's syndrome.

Subject Index